GW01605181

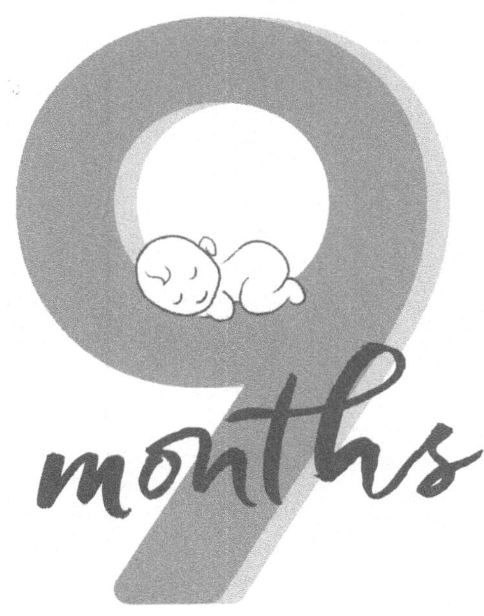
9
months

DR DAVID ADDENBROOKE
MBBS BSc(Med) BA(English) FRANZCOG
& RUBY MATLEY

9 months

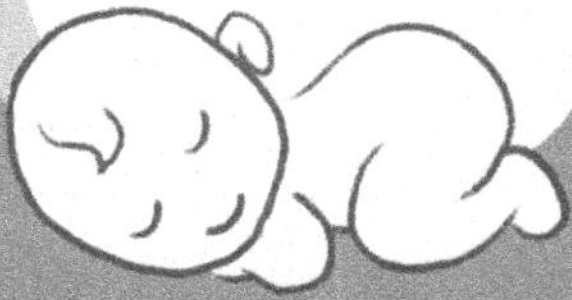

THE ESSENTIAL AUSTRALIAN GUIDE TO PREGNANCY

Pan Macmillan Australia

CONTENTS

Third Trimester 113

After the Birth 239

Recipes 257

INTRODUCTION

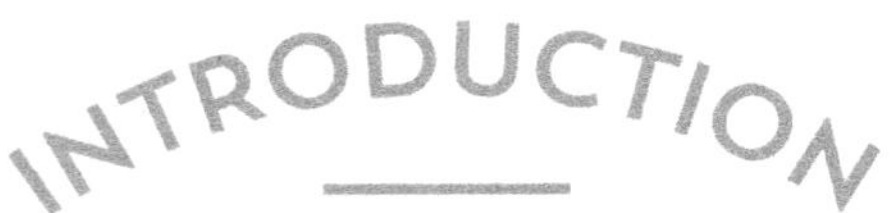

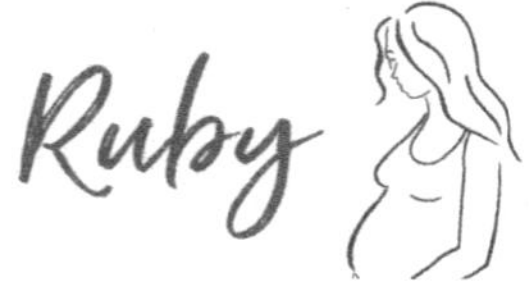

It is incredible that as women we have the ability to develop, nourish and grow another human being. It seems like yesterday that I discovered I was pregnant with my firstborn. I remember feeling scared beyond words, yet so excited at what was ahead.

Professionally speaking, I have a science degree and have worked in clinical settings. I am also curious by nature, so as soon as my pregnancy was confirmed, I set about learning everything I could. There are countless things that no one tells us when we are pregnant and many of which I wish I had known. Pregnancy, like parenthood, has a steep learning curve and there is a copious amount of information to digest. Everything is medicalised and the terminology can be confusing. I felt this even with the knowledge I already had.

So having a close friend who'd already had a child was invaluable for me. She answered all my questions, no matter how silly they seemed. I could divulge my biggest fears to her, too. With my second pregnancy, I felt more prepared, but I soon learned that every pregnancy is different and I discovered there was so much more to learn.

This is what encouraged me to write this book. I wanted to be a friend who can answer those awkward questions you may have. But I also wanted to offer the expertise of a professional. This is where David comes in.

While living in Byron Bay, I was unsure what route I wanted to take to birthing. I was somewhat hesitant to see an obstetrician, because I believed I wouldn't have my own say when it came to birthing options. This may sound a little naïve, but I had no idea what pregnancy and the birthing experience entailed.

In the end, I decided to have an obstetrician mostly because family and friends who had babies recommended it and, in hindsight, I am thankful that I did. Continuity for me was what made me feel most comfortable, reassured and supported throughout my pregnancy and postpartum period.

David's office is set in northern New South Wales. His rooms are in a large old Queenslander converted into offices that make you feel at ease as soon as you walk through the front door. After meeting David, I instantly felt comfortable, trusted and relieved. David has encyclopaedic knowledge and a soothing manner – just what I needed.

It is easy to focus on the development of the baby and forget about how you are feeling and what you may be experiencing and remembering to be kind to yourself because, after all, you are growing a human.

David and I hope that this book will answer many of the niggling questions you have about pregnancy and birth. That it will reassure you that you are not alone and that it will help you feel at ease, excited, prepared and informed about what to expect during your pregnancy.

People are connected now more than ever through the internet and social media. While these tools are excellent, they can create more anxiety, pressure and uncertainty. I hope this book enables you to trust your instincts, to celebrate all the changes that pregnancy brings, and to make informed, nurturing choices for you and your baby.

David

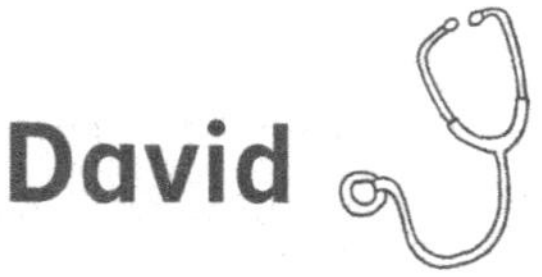

Birth never gets old.

I have been in the room for thousands of births, each with its own mix of calm, crazy and magical. On every single occasion, I have felt privileged to bear witness to these precious moments in a family's life.

I have also continued to be humbled by the gratitude expressed by women, their partners and families for the most unexpected reasons. There have been so many births in which my sole purpose was simply to be there. Often, these are the times when people feel the most thankful for their doctor or midwife, when they are simply there to encourage, empower, reassure and let birth happen.

The speciality of obstetrics is built around predicting risks, where possible, and then dealing with problems if they arise. The unfortunate result of this is that modern pregnancy has become a series of medical hurdles (or 'screening tests') and the definition of a healthy pregnancy is when the woman manages to make it through the obstacle course of investigation unscathed as a 'low risk' patient. Increasingly, women are keen to move away from the 'medicalisation of birth'. I can appreciate this sentiment.

The truth is, most women do not need a doctor to give birth. A lot of 'complications' of pregnancy and birth are more like precautions – things found by practitioners which have a chance to cause trouble, but often won't if acknowledged and treated with care. Some things that go wrong are what we call 'iatrogenic', which is a medical term roughly meaning 'the disease was caused by the treatment'. We, as doctors, need to limit these occurrences.

I've tried to write the medical sections of this book in the same way that I talk to the hundreds of women I help through pregnancy and birth each year. Where possible, I have avoided using complicated statistics or confusing scientific jargon. Everything we do in medicine is leaning towards an 'evidence-based' approach. We want you to know that the things we recommend are based on scientific research, but we also recognise that most of you aren't scientists.

This book, then, is based on experience, backed up by science, and filtered through common sense.

Importantly, however, I am not *your* obstetrician. That means that you should consult the person looking after you personally before making any decisions about what to do when you are pregnant. There often is no right way. Every woman and every birth is unique. The key to making it safer, calmer and more satisfying is having the right people around you when it happens.

Happy birthing!

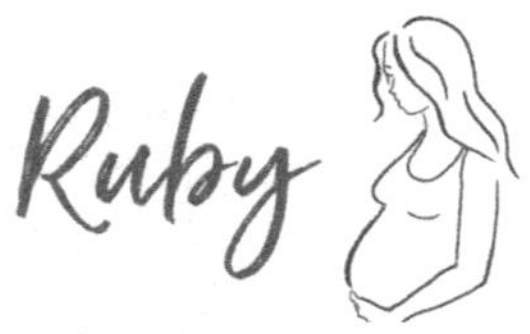

PREPARING FOR PREGNANCY

Every woman's preparation for pregnancy will be different. Some will become pregnant without time to prepare, while others will spend several months improving their health before actively trying to get pregnant. When preparing for pregnancy, the following steps are recommended:

- Start taking folic acid and iodine (see page 21) or a pregnancy supplement that contains a range of key vitamins and minerals.
- Cease or limit alcohol consumption.
- Get professional help for addictions such as smoking and drug use.
- Speak to your doctor about any medications you are taking to check whether these are safe to continue taking prior to and during pregnancy.
- Exercise regularly and eat a balanced healthy diet.

If you are overweight or obese, you may choose to seek advice and support from a doctor or dietician to reduce your weight before becoming pregnant. There is an increased risk of issues during pregnancy for women who are overweight or obese, including preeclampsia (see page 135), gestational diabetes (see page 83) and the likelihood of caesarean delivery (see page 214).

It is recommended that women have the measles, mumps and rubella (MMR) vaccination prior to becoming pregnant, as this vaccine is unable to be given during pregnancy. The vaccine guards against infections that may cause miscarriage, premature delivery or serious birth defects if you were to contract them while pregnant. If you're unsure about your immunisation history, a blood test can detect if you are protected with these antibodies.

Deciding to conceive may be the first time you've ever thought about when you're 'most fertile' or how regular your periods are, or how to spot the signs of ovulation. A period diary is a handy way to track this information, whether you jot it down on paper or use one of the many apps available. Around the time of ovulation is when we are most likely to conceive: this usually occurs around days 10–14 of a 28-day cycle, but of course your period cycle may be longer or shorter. Tracking your cycle can help you to work out when you're most fertile and therefore most likely to conceive.

Conception might be as easy as ceasing the use of contraception and tracking ovulation and next thing you know . . . you're pregnant! For some of us, though, it can be a much longer journey, involving fertility treatment, multiple miscarriages or other challenges.

A word on ART and IVF

Many pregnancy books don't touch on assisted reproduction technology (ART) and in-vitro fertilisation (IVF), usually because these are complex topics that require specialist advice and treatments. Indeed, there is an abundance of books out there that focus solely on these subjects.

You are most likely pregnant by the time you read this book; however I feel it is important to acknowledge the journey that you may have experienced to get to this point. Assisted reproduction is becoming increasingly common and, with the advancements in medicine and technologies, it is now more successful.

If you have taken the ART or IVF path, you will know firsthand the raw emotion of the ups and downs. Injections, retrievals, disappointment, anticipation and resentment may be all too familiar for both you and your partner. There can be an increased anxiety connected to pregnancy and it is common to feel more aware and cautious during each stage.

Research has shown there are links between pre- and postnatal depression and anxiety in women who have used ART. If you feel you're experiencing anxiety or depression during your pregnancy, it is important to talk about it with a health professional, family member or close friend.

David

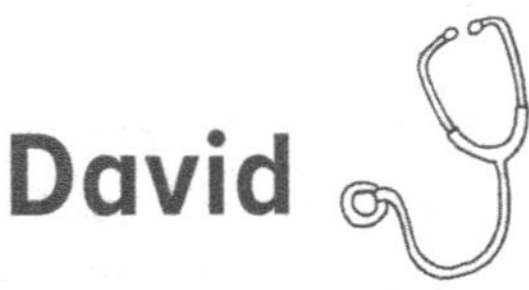

THE BASICS

Pregnancy is for 9 months, or 40 weeks. This is the average time between the start of your last menstrual period and the time a baby is born.

Strangely enough, you are not actually pregnant for the first 2 weeks of gestation. Ovulation occurs, on average, 14–16 days after the first day of a period. This is the first opportunity for the sperm to fertilise the egg, so conception doesn't occur until around this time. Even after an egg is fertilised, it doesn't actually implant into your womb for another week. For up to 9 days, the fertilised egg, or embryo, is floating in your womb or tubes, growing and getting ready to attach. Your own body is not even aware that a pregnancy has occurred until a few days before your period is due.

The typical conception rate for couples of all ages when actively trying to fall pregnant is about 20 per cent per menstrual cycle. The rate is higher for younger couples and lower for older couples.

There are basically three parts (trimesters) of a pregnancy. Conveniently, these last about 3 months each.

1 – The first trimester (weeks 1 to 12) is all about your body starting to recognise that you are pregnant, with major hormonal changes that can lead to fatigue and feelings of nausea. Changes in the way your body deals with distribution of your blood to your uterus can increase your heart rate or reduce your blood pressure. Ligaments begin to soften and bones shift. Your body is gearing up to make nutrients available to create another person, and your tummy is going to need to make space to grow it.

2 – The second trimester (weeks 13 to 26) is about making sure the baby is developing normally and growing big enough so that it can survive outside the womb. This is the bit where you get to post the picture of the baby from the ultrasound, but you might not really feel all that pregnant yet – maybe even less pregnant if the morning sickness has settled. At some point you will develop a 'bump' and feel those magical first kicks. I call this the 'honeymoon period'

because your body has hopefully settled in to a lot of the hormonal and physiological changes that occurred in the first trimester, but your baby is still not big enough to put too much pressure on your pelvis and diaphragm.

3 – The third trimester is week 27 to birth. The baby starts stacking on weight, gets in the right position and fine-tunes the last little tweaks on the organ systems to enable life. This is the time when everybody asks you when you are due as the birth is starting to draw closer.

There is also a fourth part – the point where baby is totally able to survive outside the womb without anybody worrying about prematurity. Luckily, this part doesn't last for 3 months, but it is variable and can last over a month. This is called 'full term' and is anywhere from 37 to 42 weeks, and beyond. The 'due date' is at exactly 40 weeks, but this is just a convenient number that falls in the middle of this large range of dates in which it would be completely normal for your birth to happen.

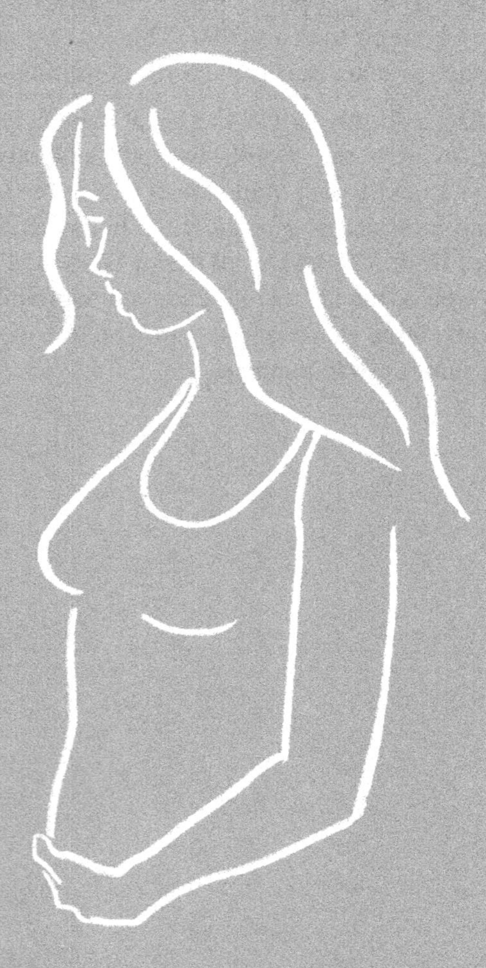

FIRST TRIMESTER

David 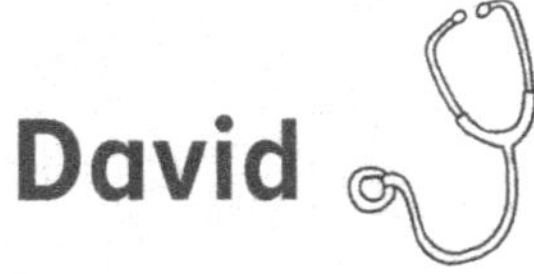

The first trimester can be a bit of a 3-month mind game for some mothers. You know you are pregnant but you can't really feel anything in there yet. You may be happy or scared or surprised that this has happened – or maybe a mix of all three. There may also be a part of you that doesn't want to get too excited yet, because you know there is a chance that things may not go to plan. All of these reactions are normal.

Meanwhile, your body is getting on with it. You may feel very tired and nauseous, and find that you vomit at any time of the day or night. (I have been corrected on numerous occasions by my patients who remind me it is not 'morning sickness', but 'all-day sickness'.) You may feel bloated and/or constipated. Your heart will be beating faster than usual. You may already start to notice changes in your skin and hair. That 'pregnancy glow' is your capillaries dilating in response to the hormonal changes.

During the early stages of pregnancy, your baby's brain, spine, neural tissues and central nervous system begin to form. The heart and organs start to develop by the end of the first trimester. The embryo will develop into a fetus over the coming weeks, and his or her little fingers, toes and eyes will begin to take shape.

The pregnancy hormone, hCG

You may hear your doctor mention hCG, or spot it on your pathology paperwork. HCG stands for human chorionic gonadotropin, otherwise known as the pregnancy hormone. HCG is what is detected when you use an at-home pregnancy test. The hormone is produced by the placenta and increases in the first trimester. It is detected in the urine, which is why your pregnancy test shows positive.

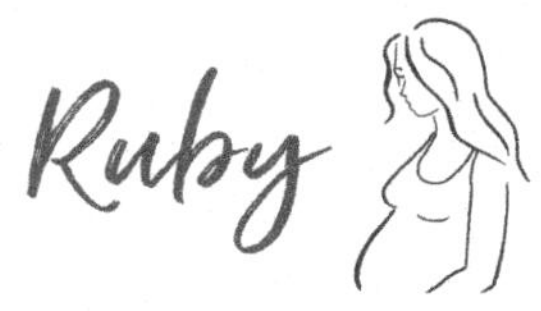

EARLY SIGNS OF PREGNANCY

The absence of a period is the first firm sign of pregnancy for most women. But you may experience symptoms before you have discovered you've missed a period. These include:

- spotting
- abdominal cramping
- breast changes, including tenderness and enlargement
- fatigue
- nausea or vomiting ('morning sickness'; see page 46)
- changes in mood
- passing urine more frequently.

Many symptoms experienced in the first trimester, such as fatigue and morning sickness, should subside as the pregnancy progresses, although some of the symptoms can stick around for longer and, in some cases, last the entire pregnancy.

What I'm really thinking . . .

Two little lines

Once you see those two lines on the home pregnancy test, life changes. When I found out I was pregnant for the first time, my initial reaction was a mix of joyful excitement and nervousness. I remember thinking, *Am I going to be able to do this? What will it be like to be pregnant? How is it going to change my life?*

After discovering I was pregnant for the second time, I felt ecstatic but I was also consumed by worry. My daughter had only just turned 1 and I questioned whether I was going to be able to look after two little people and give them the love and attention they deserved.

On both occasions, I felt delighted and anxious at the same time. I know now that these feelings are a completely normal response to such a life-changing moment – and just the start of an incredibly emotional journey.

David

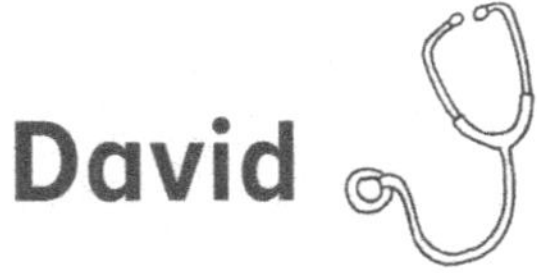

YOU'RE PREGNANT: WHAT NEXT?

Write down the first day of your last period. This will help you and your healthcare provider figure out exactly how far along you are. The important date is the first day that you bled with your last period. Don't worry if you can't remember exactly – it just means your doctor will have to rely a little more on an ultrasound to work out your baby's due date.

Start taking a pregnancy multivitamin. The most vital component to be taking as early as possible is folic acid, the synthetic form of folate (vitamin B9). This helps development of the baby's brain and spinal cord, which happens as early as 4 weeks in. Most pregnancy supplements contain the recommended doses of other important vitamins and minerals, such as vitamin D, iodine, calcium and iron. Some of the minerals can be hard to digest and contribute to nausea and/or constipation. If this is the case, try taking a folic acid tablet on its own at least until you are able to digest the full multi. See page 21 for more on supplements.

Stop drinking alcohol. As there is no evidence for a 'safe' amount of alcohol in pregnancy, doctors advise complete abstinence. If you are planning to fall pregnant, it is best to stop before you start trying. Don't panic if you unexpectedly conceive during a time when you'd been drinking or if you had a few drinks in the days before you knew you were pregnant. Unintentional alcohol exposure in the first trimester does increase your chance of a miscarriage, but if you stop as soon as you find out, it is unlikely your baby will suffer any long-term effects. Most data on drinking while pregnant comes from chronic or heavy use later in pregnancy.

If you smoke, reduce then stop your nicotine intake. Smoking while pregnant causes damage to the placenta, which is basically doing all of the work for the baby's lungs, kidneys and intestines while it is in your womb. This damage increases your risk of all sorts of bad things happening during pregnancy and is associated with lower birth rates. A smaller baby due to an unhealthy placenta has an increased risk of stillbirth, separation of the placenta (called abruption), or not tolerating labour leading to a higher chance of caesarean birth. Smoking is also, obviously, bad for you. While nicotine replacement is not accepted as 'safe' in pregnancy, it is almost certainly better than smoking tobacco. If you can stop cold turkey, all the better – and you will certainly have an excellent motivation.

If you take prescription medication, talk with your doctor. Some medications are known to cause birth defects. There are others that may have small acceptable risks but need further discussion with your doctor depending on your condition. There are many prescription drugs that are perfectly safe to take while pregnant. It is important that you don't stop your meds without having discussed it with your doctor. This is particularly true for medications used in conditions such as epilepsy and depression, some of which can have negative effects on your baby but which may also have severe effects for the mother if stopped abruptly.

If you have a chronic illness, see your doctor. Many illnesses can be affected by pregnancy, including diabetes, high blood pressure, thyroid disorders, epilepsy, blood clotting disorders, auto-immune conditions and mood disorders. Ideally you would discuss management of these conditions before getting pregnant.

Tell the people you are comfortable telling. A pregnancy is a very personal and private thing for you and your partner. There are no right or wrong answers about who to tell, just whatever feels right to you. The reason many people wait until after 12 weeks is because of the higher rate of pregnancies that fail in this time. Across all women in all age groups, roughly 1 in 5 pregnancies will not continue past the first trimester. There are many factors that influence this, one of which is age. The miscarriage rate for a woman in her early 20s is around 1 in 10, while that of a woman in her 40s can be higher than 1 in 2. Whilst a pregnancy is a private experience, a miscarriage can be even more so. In the case of an early pregnancy loss, having someone to share your feelings with can be important.

See a doctor or midwife. In addition to helping you plan the rest of the pregnancy and birth, seeing a doctor or midwife in the first trimester is important to start some screening tests. There are a number of blood tests that all pregnant women are routinely advised to have. Some tests are relevant to all women, such as knowing your blood group and making sure you are not anaemic. Most doctors recommend additional screening for some infectious diseases that can impact on the developing baby. A lot of these, such as HIV, are fairly uncommon in Australia; however this is particularly important for women who have recently been living in high-risk countries or situations. Many doctors also check for additional nutritional factors, such as vitamin D stores, or carry out baseline organ function tests such as liver, kidney and thyroid. You can also have an initial discussion about how and where you want to have your baby.

Consider getting an ultrasound. These days, most couples tend to associate the first ultrasound with confirmation that they are really, truly pregnant. There is definitely something validating and powerful about seeing the heartbeat flickering on the screen. For many, it is the moment when it becomes *real*. However, it is not something that is absolutely required in the first trimester.

Live your life. When it comes to normal day-to-day physical activity, there is nothing you should or shouldn't be doing. It is perfectly safe to exercise, swim, work and have sex when you are in the early stages of a pregnancy. Studies have shown that women who spend the first trimester on strict bed rest are no more or less likely to miscarry than women undertaking normal activities. However, women on strict bed rest were more likely to develop other negative physical or emotional effects, such as depression or blood clots in the legs.

Calculating your due date

If you have a regular 28-day cycle, you can calculate your due date by adding 40 weeks to the first day of your last period. This is exactly what that wheel you see midwives and obstetricians using does. Of course, many patients and clinicians now use apps and websites. Keep in mind some factors may make a due date based on your period inaccurate, such as if you have an unpredictable cycle or have just come off hormonal contraception.

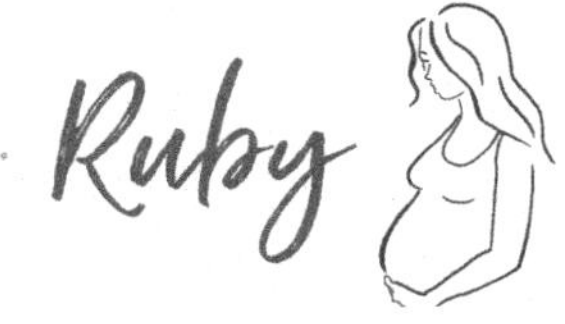

SELF-CARE IN THE FIRST TRIMESTER

For many women, the first trimester can appear to crawl along at a snail's pace when all they want is for it to pass quickly, not only to leave the early nausea and fatigue behind, but also to reach the 12-week mark (at which point the pregnancy is generally considered to be 'safe'). The first trimester can be draining for these reasons, so it is a time to be kind and gentle to yourself. Aim to do things that will help reduce your stress levels, and if that means lying on the sofa and reading a book or watching a movie, then do it! Allow yourself to rest if you are feeling fatigued and be sure to nourish your body with healthy food. Here are some ideas for 'you time':

- Read. It doesn't have to be pregnancy or parenting related; there is nothing better than getting lost in a book for a while and escaping from everyday worries.
- Listen to calming music.
- Go for a long walk in the park.
- Start a pregnancy journal. You could jot down questions or concerns you may be having, how you are feeling or even possible baby names. Your journal could be something you look back on down the track to remember your pregnancy.

And some things your partner can do:

- Make cups of ginger tea, to help ease any nausea.
- Encourage rest.
- Go along to the antenatal appointments, if possible.
- Be positive and validate what your partner is experiencing. She may experience mood changes throughout pregnancy, particularly in the early months when her body is changing and hormones are fluctuating.

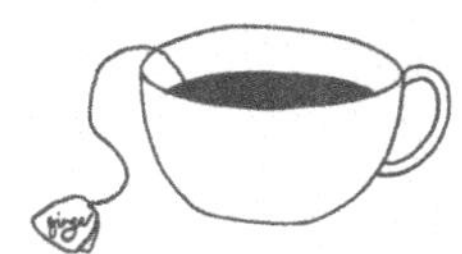

What I'm really thinking . . .

The early weeks

I was so unbelievably happy when I found out I was pregnant, yet so nervous at the same time. I felt a little overwhelmed about holding this big secret, knowing that I still had another 8 weeks of keeping it quiet. (I felt that not sharing the news until we were over the 12-week hurdle was the best option for me.) 'Don't get your hopes up, don't get too excited,' I kept telling myself. Realistically, though, from the moment I discovered I was pregnant, I started to envisage life with this little being. I calculated the due date and kept it close to my heart.

I experienced such a mix of emotions in those early weeks – excitement, love, empowerment, nervousness and disbelief. I was also horrifically nauseous. I kept crackers by my bed and had ginger tea constantly brewing to give me some relief, because the nausea seemed to linger for weeks. I felt anxious and had moments where my heart would race: I still don't know if it was the hormones or the waiting game. I was bloated and felt uncomfortable. Around the 7-week mark, the fatigue kicked in and I had a little bit of spotting that lasted around a week.

Throughout the first trimester, you may also have moments when you are feel vulnerable or anxious. But you may also experience times when you are full of love and gratitude, as you embrace the changes to come and the excitement of growing your baby.

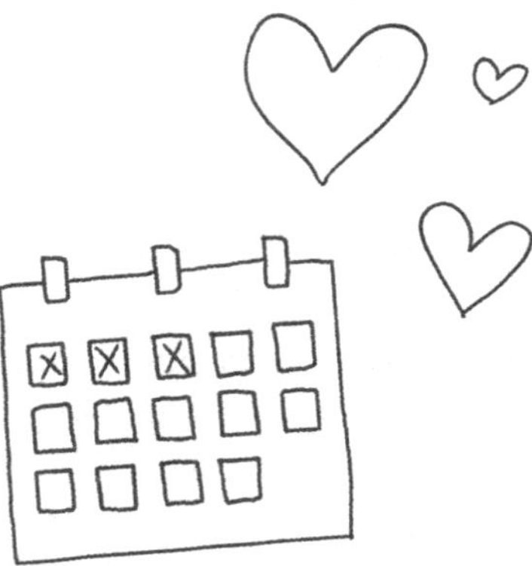

EATING WELL

Over the next 9 months, your body has an incredibly important job to do, and your baby will need a range of nutrients for healthy growth and development. Eating well is paramount, but there is no need to follow any strict diets. The aim is to nourish your body and your baby without limiting food groups.

Try not to worry if you are unable to follow the 'ideal' pregnancy diet due to feeling nauseous or vomiting. I remember asking David whether my baby would be at risk if I was not eating the 'perfect' food all the time. He put my mind at ease by explaining that babies are like parasites and they take the nutrients from you first!

We all get busy and sometimes the easy option is to eat on the run. Here are a few tips to ensure you eat well during pregnancy:

- Prepare meals over the weekend for the following week, so that you are less likely to eat out and potentially choose unhealthy options.

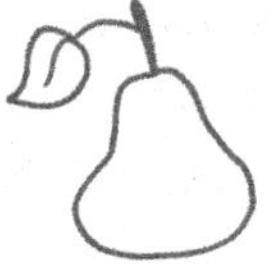

- Make larger quantities of healthy meals at dinnertime and store them in the freezer for a later date.
- Keep nutritious snacks at work or with you during the day (see page 23).

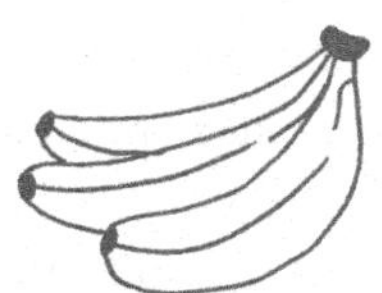

- Prepare a vegetarian meal once or twice a week to incorporate eggs, legumes and more vegetables into your diet.

And of course you're allowed to indulge from time to time – after all, you are pregnant!

YOUR DAILY PLATE

During your pregnancy, it is recommended that you increase your consumption of whole grains, vegetables, protein and dairy foods to ensure that you and your baby receive adequate nutrients, minerals and vitamins.

In addition, it is best to always choose foods that are nutrient-dense rather than high in calories. Avoid processed foods as much as possible, and try to limit your intake of items high in sugar, such as soft drinks. It is also recommended that you reduce your intake of saturated fats, especially trans fats (which are typically found in packaged and processed foods).

Protein

Protein is found in lean meat, chicken, seafood, eggs, dairy products, nuts and legumes. It is crucial for your baby's growth and development, particularly during the third trimester. Many protein-rich foods are also high in B vitamins (especially B12) and healthy fats. Eating protein will also assist in feeling satisfied after meals.

Grains, legumes, nuts and seeds

Whole grains (such as brown rice, quinoa, buckwheat and oats) and beans, peas and lentils help to maintain steady blood sugar levels and are rich in fibre, which is beneficial for your bowel and particularly good if you are suffering from constipation. Almonds, cashews, walnuts, peanuts, sunflower seeds and sesame seeds are all excellent sources of fibre and healthy fats.

Vegetables

Vegetables are truly great for your health. They are rich in vitamins and minerals, and most are high in fibre. It is really important that you try to eat an abundance of different vegetables during pregnancy. The great thing about them is that they can be prepared in so many ways: you can roast root veggies such as carrot, pumpkin, sweet potato and beetroot; stir-fry green leafy vegetables such as broccoli, kale, spinach and Asian vegetables; create a salad of lettuce, avocado, tomato, cucumber and capsicum, or try some of my recipe ideas on pages 257–69.

Fruit

Fruit is high in antioxidants and nutrients such as vitamin C, potassium and folate. Fruit also contains fibre, which will help if you are suffering from constipation.

Dairy

Dairy products, including yoghurt, milk and cheese, are high in calcium. They are also good sources of B vitamins, protein and healthy fat.

ESSENTIAL VITAMINS AND MINERALS

Iron

Iron is vital for your baby's growth. Most pregnancy multivitamins contain iron; however, eating iron-rich foods can also assist in maintaining healthy stores during pregnancy and prevent anaemia. Animal sources of iron are absorbed most efficiently and include lean beef, lamb, chicken, pork, fish and seafood. Plant-based sources include beans, lentils, chickpeas, tofu and nuts. Vitamin C plays a key role in absorption of iron in the body, so try squeezing lemon juice over your spinach or drinking orange juice with meals.

If you are vegan or vegetarian, it is highly likely your GP, midwife or obstetrician will recommend having bloods taken to check if you need iron supplementation throughout your pregnancy. These blood tests may be repeated later in pregnancy to ensure you are not anaemic. The Royal Australian and New Zealand College of Obstetrics and Gynaecology (RANZCOG) suggests women with iron deficiency take at least 60 mg of iron daily during pregnancy.

Calcium

Calcium is important for healthy bones and teeth and is vital during pregnancy. Vitamin D aids in the absorption of calcium. Calcium-rich foods, including milk, cheese and yoghurt, are also sources of vitamin B12, which is important for your baby's neurological development and metabolic health. Yoghurt also contains lactobacillus cultures, which can aid digestion if you are lactose intolerant. If you have a cow's milk allergy, you can drink calcium-fortified non-dairy milks. Other good sources of calcium include salmon, sardines, tofu, nuts, seeds and dark green leafy vegetables.

Zinc

Zinc is essential for normal fetal development. Research has shown links between low zinc intake during pregnancy and issues with immunological development, growth and congenital abnormalities. Most prenatal vitamin supplements contain zinc. Beef, lamb, pork, chicken and fish contain the highest levels of zinc, although beans, pumpkin seeds, eggs and dairy products are also good sources.

Vitamin B12

Vitamin B12 in pregnancy is essential for the healthy development of your baby's central nervous system. Your pregnancy multivitamin most likely contains the recommended amount, but you can also increase your intake by eating foods rich in vitamin B12 such as milk, dairy products and eggs.

Vitamin D

We mostly get our vitamin D from sunlight; however, you can also take it as a supplement. Sun exposure during pregnancy is not only good for your immune function and bone health but also beneficial for your baby, so it is a great idea to get out into the sunshine every day, even if it is only for a few minutes. Remember, of course, to stay sun smart and avoid going out during the hottest part of the day. Calcium (see page 19) helps the body to absorb vitamin D.

What supplements should I take?

Folate (vitamin B9) is known as **folic acid** in its synthetic form. Scientific research has shown that adequate folate intake during pregnancy reduces the risk of neural tube defects (NTD) in babies, which lead to spina bifida and anencephaly. Folate can be found in fortified foods such as bread and cereals. Most pregnancy or prenatal vitamins will also contain it. The daily dose recommended by RANZCOG is at least 0.4 mg to aid the prevention of neural tube defects.

Iodine is an essential trace mineral that our bodies need to make thyroid hormones. During pregnancy iodine plays a vital role in your baby's brain and nervous system development. Iodine can be found in seafood and seaweed products, as well as milk, cheese and yoghurt. It can also be found in fish, some fruits and vegetables and iodised salt. RANZCOG recommends that women who are pregnant, breastfeeding or planning to become pregnant should take an iodine supplement of 150 mcg daily. Most, if not all, pregnancy multivitamins have iodine in them – check the ingredients list.

Omega-3 fatty acids are particularly important for fetal brain development and the healthy development of the retina. The best food source of omega-3 fatty acids is oily fish, such as sardines and wild-caught salmon.

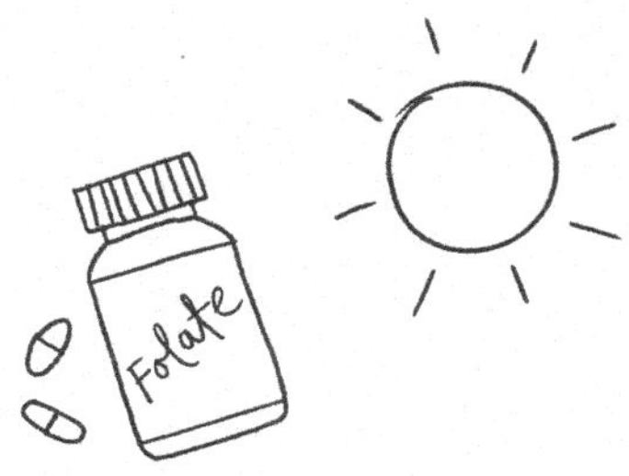

What I'm really thinking . . .

Eating healthily

When I became pregnant, my goal was to nourish my body by eating a wide variety of foods but still enjoy the occasional treat, especially chocolate! In reality, in the first trimester I couldn't stomach much of anything other than toast and herbal tea. As the nausea subsided, I started to get more creative with my cooking. I also tried out healthy snacks (see opposite). Some days I was ravenous and seemed to be constantly seeking out my next meal.

At times the lists of what I 'should' and 'shouldn't' be eating felt overwhelming. I worried that my baby wasn't getting all the nutrients it needed – especially when some days all I felt like eating were chicken schnitzel and ice blocks! Taking a pregnancy supplement helped to ease my mind, as did planning my meals to ensure all food groups were covered. I found that it was best to keep things simple: there was no need to spend lots of money on special ingredients or 'superfoods'. And I also learned to give myself a break. If I really felt like something, I ate it (as long as it was safe). Everything in moderation.

Should I be eating for two?

You may feel hungrier than usual and have certain food preferences during pregnancy, both of which are okay. There is no need to double your intake of food, though. Nutrients including calcium, protein, iron and folate play vital roles in the growth and development of your baby, but eating a diet that is nutrient-dense, rather than larger quantities of food, will ensure you receive adequate amounts of nutrients.

Dealing with food allergies

If you have a diagnosed allergy, you should continue to avoid allergenic foods while pregnant. Otherwise, there is no need to avoid allergens such as tree nuts, dairy and eggs while pregnant or breastfeeding. No sufficient evidence exists to suggest that avoiding food allergens while pregnant will decrease your baby's risk of developing a food allergy.

IDEAS FOR HEALTHY SNACKS & MEALS

- Handfuls of nuts and seeds. I love to roast pumpkin seeds with a splash of tamari for an easy, on-the-go snack.
- Keep your fruit bowl stocked with a range of fresh fruit. Poach any apples that are looking a little brown and serve them with a dollop of Greek yoghurt.
- Eggs. Remember to cook them well or ask for well done if you're dining out.
- Greek yoghurt served with fruit and a sprinkle of seeds and almond meal is quick, easy and nutritious.
- Whole grain crackers or bread with avocado or cheese.
- Hummus with vegetable sticks.
- Frozen edamame (soybeans) are great to have on hand.
- Whole grain toasted sandwich filled with cheese, avocado, tomato and baby spinach.
- Tuna or chicken salad with lots of vegetables makes a perfect light dinner, especially in the later months of pregnancy when you don't feel like a big meal.
- And see pages 257–69 for more ideas.

FOOD SAFETY IN PREGNANCY

Food safety during pregnancy is important, but should not be something that makes you feel anxious. Taking some simple precautions will help to reduce the risks and keep you and your baby safe.

Food-borne illnesses such as listeria and salmonella may require treatment with antibiotics, as well as support for the mother with hydration and fever management.

Toxoplasmosis

Toxoplasmosis is an infection caused by the parasite *Toxoplasma gondii*. It is important that women take precautions to not contract the infection while pregnant, as the parasite can affect the unborn baby if it crosses the placenta.

Take these steps to avoid toxoplasmosis:

- Wash your hands after touching raw meat.
- Cook meat thoroughly; avoid rare or medium–rare meat.
- Wear gloves while gardening.
- If you have a cat, ask someone else to handle the litter tray and ensure it is cleaned daily.

Salmonella

Salmonella is a bacterium linked to food poisoning. We can become infected with it by ingesting contaminated food and water, which may cause symptoms such as vomiting, nausea, cramps, diarrhoea and fever. Chicken and eggs are the most likely sources of salmonella.

To reduce your risk of infection:

- Make sure chicken is always thoroughly cooked.
- Don't eat raw or soft-cooked eggs.
- Avoid raw fish and shellfish, such as sushi and sashimi, and oysters.

Listeria

Caused by the bacteria *Listeria monocytogenes*, listeriosis is a rare infection that can be passed from a pregnant woman to her unborn baby. It can be contracted through uncooked food or foods that haven't been stored or handled correctly. Symptoms may include muscle aches, headache, nausea, diarrhoea, fever, drowsiness and confusion. Treatment requires hospitalisation and intravenous antibiotics.

Take the following precautions to reduce your risk of infection:

- Avoid unpasteurised dairy products, raw seafood and soft-serve ice cream.
- Wash vegetables and fruit thoroughly.
- Store and handle food correctly and carefully: keep fresh produce in the fridge, always check use-by and best-before dates, heat food to the correct temperature, and wash your hands thoroughly before preparing meals.

FOOD CRAVINGS AND AVERSIONS

Food cravings and aversions are relatively common during pregnancy. All I yearned for during the first few months of my pregnancy was sauerkraut, pickles and citrus fruits. The cravings started to settle down around 5–6 months, although there were certainly times in the later months when requests for strawberries and liquorice were high on the list. Towards the end of the pregnancy, I 'emotionally' ate, seeking foods that contained sugar. I blame this on fatigue and the need for a pick-me-up in the afternoon.

You may have heard of pica, which is the persistent craving to ingest a non-food substance such as dirt, clay, paper or chalk. Although pica isn't common during pregnancy, if you have these cravings it is important not to consume these substances as a health precaution, and to speak with your midwife or doctor.

WHAT SHOULD I AVOID?

Alcohol

There is so much confusion around alcohol consumption during pregnancy, particularly when it comes to low-level drinking such as having the odd drink for special occasions. Be prepared for your friends and family members to all have different opinions on the matter, but you must make the decision you are comfortable with. Importantly, research has not been able to identify a safe level of alcohol consumption during pregnancy. The Australian Institute of Health and Welfare guidelines recommend that pregnant women avoid alcohol completely. Heavy alcohol consumption during pregnancy is harmful for a developing fetus and can lead to fetal alcohol spectrum disorders ranging from behavioural and developmental issues to severe, lifelong physical impairments.

Cigarettes

Smoking has adverse effects on the fetus. If you are a smoker, quitting prior to becoming pregnant or in early pregnancy will give your baby the best start to life. Smoking while pregnant increases the risk of miscarriage and stillbirth. Carbon monoxide, nicotine and other poisons contained in cigarettes are passed directly to your baby via your bloodstream. There are several quit-smoking programs available that can assist you.

Caffeine

The great news is that you don't have to give up your morning coffee! However, caffeine should be consumed in moderation. The guidelines recommend pregnant women consume no more than 200 mg of caffeine per day. To put it in perspective, that is equivalent to 1 cup of strong coffee or about 3 cups of black tea. It is important to note that energy drinks, chocolate and other products contain caffeine, so you may need to limit these too. There is no research to suggest that consuming caffeine during pregnancy causes birth defects.

Raw fish

It is recommended that pregnant women avoid eating raw fish such as sushi, sashimi and oysters (as well as raw eggs and undercooked meats) due to the increased risk of food-borne illnesses.

Unpasteurised dairy products

Unpasteurised milk and soft cheeses, such as camembert and blue cheese, are more likely to be contaminated with listeria if not properly handled or stored. The good news is most of the cheeses we purchase from the supermarket are pasteurised and if you store and handle them correctly at home, this makes the risk considerably low. Be sure to consume these products in moderation and purchase them from a reputable store or supermarket.

Feta cheese, if store-bought, is very low risk and safe for pregnant women to consume. Other cheeses that are safe to consume during pregnancy include cream cheese, haloumi, cheddar, parmesan and other hard cheeses.

Some beauty products

A few ingredients found in beauty products should be avoided during pregnancy. These include the following:

Vitamin A (retinol): A lot of anti-aging cosmetics, acne creams and some sunscreens contain retinol, a vitamin A formula that may be harmful to use. Research has shown that vitamin A taken orally during pregnancy can cause major birth defects. Although there has been some research on the skin absorption levels of topical vitamin A, there is not enough research specific to pregnant women to be sure it is safe. Therefore, most health professionals will suggest that pregnant women avoid using retinol/vitamin A-based cosmetics. It is a good idea to read through the ingredients in your bathroom cabinet to check if any of your usual cosmetics contain vitamin A or retinol, just to be on the safe side.

Hydnoquinone: Hydnoquinone is a skin-whitening agent used to treat melasma (darkening of the pigment in the skin that can occur during pregnancy). However, it should not be used during pregnancy. Dermatologists recommend you wait until after you have ceased breastfeeding before using hydnoquinone as the absorption rate through the skin is high.

Botox: When it comes to anti-aging treatments such as Botox or fillers, it is advised that you do not have these done while you are pregnant, as there is not enough medical research into their effects.

Saunas and steam rooms

Obstetric guidelines recommend that pregnant women avoid using saunas and steam rooms. This is also the case with very hot baths (baths that are painfully hot and make your skin turn pink). The guidelines don't specify an exact temperature range, but a comfortably warm bath is perfectly safe and a great way for you to relax (you'll appreciate a bath as your growing bump gets bigger and you begin to get aches and pains!).

Can I still dye my hair?

Many women stop dyeing their hair during pregnancy and it is very much a personal decision. There is no scientific evidence to suggest that using hair dye during pregnancy will cause any harm to your unborn baby. However, just to be on the safe side, you may wish to wait until week 12 of pregnancy before dyeing your hair. If you are exposed occupationally (if you are a hairdresser or beauty therapist), it is a good idea to reduce your exposure by using safety measures such as wearing gloves, having good ventilation and safeguarding storage and disposal of chemicals.

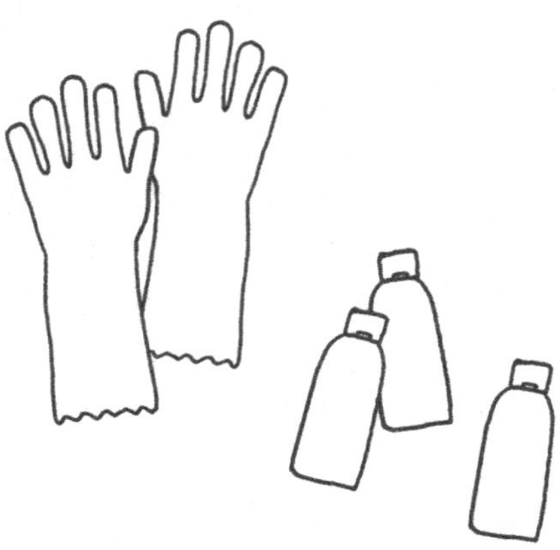

ANTENATAL CARE

In Australia, there are a number of paths you can take when it comes to antenatal care and birthing your baby. It is a good idea to explore your options and choose the care that feels most right for you and your baby, depending on your specific requirements and outlook. This could be a private obstetrician, a midwife-led birth centre or a shared-care arrangement with your GP. The important thing is to find a person or team who you trust, and who will support your pregnancy and birth choices.

If you are a public patient, you will first visit your GP, who will take care of all the necessary blood tests, screenings and vaccinations you may need, and also arrange referrals to health specialists should you need to see them. You will visit the antenatal outpatient clinic at your nearest public hospital from around the 12-week mark. Regular check-ups will be done through the outpatient service, primarily with midwives. You may also see an obstetrician if there are any complications or concerns (such as breech birth).

If you are a patient with private health insurance, or a self-funded patient choosing to have an obstetrician, you will receive a referral from your GP, and then see your obstetrician for the duration of your pregnancy. You may decide to give birth in a private hospital, or in a public hospital as a private patient, with a private obstetrician of your choice.

It can be a strange task finding the right obstetrician for you. Ask friends, family members and colleagues if they have any recommendations. Or maybe you're lucky and already have a gynaecologist who you trust. If not, start by doing your research. Look online and contact their rooms to ask about fees and waitlists, which hospitals they work out of and whether they are taking on new patients. Often meeting an obstetrician in person is the best way to decide whether they are right for you.

If you want to have the obstetrician of your choice but don't have private health insurance, you can be a self-funded patient. This means you can give birth in a public hospital but will be required to pay any out-of-pocket expenses yourself, straight to the obstetrician.

Depending on the facilities available at your hospital, you may be able to choose to either go through a birth centre or a midwife clinic.

To go through the birth centre, your pregnancy must be 'low-risk', which means if you're pregnant with multiples or have any conditions or complications, this may not be an option for you. Birthing centres are run primarily by midwives for women who are choosing to have a natural birth with minimal intervention. If you require an epidural or C-section, you will be transferred to the nearest hospital (or ward in the same hospital) that has the necessary medical equipment and facilities.

With midwife care, midwives will meet with you at scheduled intervals throughout your pregnancy, usually starting around 12 weeks onwards. They will provide you with guidance and advice on pregnancy and birthing options. Some public teaching hospitals have what they call a caseload, or midwife care program (see page 32). This is one-on-one care in which you see one midwife for the duration of your pregnancy. This continuity of care provides reassurance and support and helps to build self-confidence, which can reduce anxiety and empower you throughout your pregnancy. When you contact your local hospital, ask if this is an option.

If you have a GP who you trust and who knows you well, you may choose to have GP shared-care arrangement with the hospital. This means that you will have regular check-ups with your GP and routine appointments with the midwives. Some women like to take this path as they already have an established relationship with their GP and feel more comfortable having their support and guidance throughout the pregnancy.

David

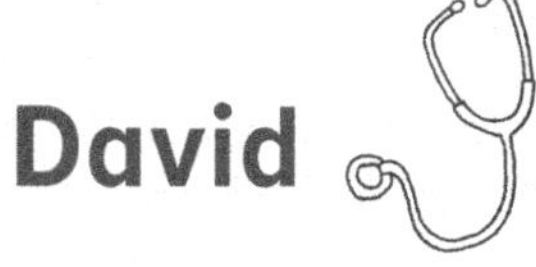

YOUR PREGNANCY TEAM

In a perfect system, 'continuity of care' should involve the whole team of GP, midwife and obstetrician.

The GP

This is often the first person you will see after a positive pregnancy test. If you have a regular GP, they will have a good idea about your general health and any things to be careful of in pregnancy for you in particular. A GP referral is also needed to access a lot of the care options available for pregnancy, as well as some of the initial tests. Many GPs have a lot of experience in managing pregnancy, and some even deliver babies regularly (often referred to as GP Obstetricians). When the GP is involved in your care throughout the pregnancy, this is called 'GP shared care'.

GP Obstetricians are more common in rural and remote areas. These doctors are mainly trained as general practitioners but have a special interest in obstetrics without having completed full training as a specialist. Some of them have a huge amount of experience, and have usually done at least a year of additional training in a hospital with specialist obstetricians.

Even if they won't be at your birth, your GP remains a valuable member of the team looking after you. In particular, their more general focus gives them a bigger picture of your health. They can help pull together advice from multiple specialists and care providers who might be involved if you have additional health challenges.

Midwives

Midwives form a core part of the staff in hospital maternity units. In Australian public hospitals, midwives do most of the straight-forward births. The notion of midwives being 'nurses who deliver babies' is a false one though. Midwifery has become quite distinct to nursing, and most newly qualified midwives actually have no nursing background at all.

Increasingly, midwives are becoming independent practitioners. Some are now able to offer full care for women with low-risk pregnancies from beginning to end. Midwives often have a very holistic view of pregnancy and childbirth. A lot of independent midwives have a more 'glass half-full' approach to pregnancy management, with a focus on the normal. Doctors can sometimes fall into the trap of a 'glass half-empty' approach, by keeping the focus on risks. Indeed, the first visit with an obstetrician is commonly referred to as a 'risk assessment'.

There are many models of care that midwives are involved in. Most hospital-employed midwives work on 8–10 hour shifts, so that during the course of labour, it is not unusual to be cared for by two or three different midwives. Over the last couple of decades, many caseload midwifery units have been developed in Australian hospitals. These midwives often work in the units referred to as birth centres. The core philosophy of these units is to try to keep the same midwife (or small group of midwives) involved from beginning to end. This principle of 'continuity of care' is an important one in pregnancy management, as it has consistently been proven to give better outcomes for women and their babies. This continuity may be from a midwife, GP or obstetrician. The development of trust and consistency of advice is thought to be where a lot of the benefit lies.

Unfortunately, when difficulties arise during a pregnancy or labour, midwife continuity sometimes has to defer to medical care. Midwives in Australia do not deliver babies by vacuum, forceps or caesarean section. If an assisted birth is required, this is one circumstance when midwives will ask an obstetrician or other hospital doctor to attend. All registered midwives in Australia are required to have the facility to access medical advice and care for women who fall outside of strict guidelines during the course of their pregnancy as well. This is a common source of disappointment for some women, when they become excluded from midwifery-led care.

Even if you have a private obstetrician, midwives will usually still be involved in monitoring you during labour and are able to manage a wide variety of emergency situations if the need arises.

Obstetricians

Obstetricians are able to manage the full spectrum of pregnancies and births, from the perfectly normal through to those with serious complications. As mentioned, obstetric training does have a focus on risk minimisation, which sometimes requires medical intervention. As a colleague once said to me, a good obstetrician knows when to intervene, and when to 'sit on their hands'.

One of the greatest rewards in private practice is the fact that most pregnancies and births I manage are 'normal'. This is a bit of a contrast to my training in public hospitals, where usually the doctor is only called when things are no longer 'normal'. As a trainee, it felt like a typical day if I introduced myself to a couple only moments before performing an emergency forceps delivery of the baby. In contrast, when I have got to know a couple over the 6 to 9 months prior, we have developed mutual trust and an understanding of birth goals.

A good obstetrician will be able to see you through everything your pregnancy or birth can throw at them, no matter what. A good obstetrician should also not intervene just for the sake of it.

Hospital doctors

While it is true that obstetricians and GPs work in hospitals and do a lot of the patient care for pregnant women, there is a lot of variation in the experience and skill level of doctors staffing maternity units in Australian public hospitals. I have listed a few of the doctor types that you may come across as a patient in an Australian hospital to make it easier to understand where they fit into your care, and what background and experience they may have.

Intern – This is a doctor who has been out of medical school for less than a year. Interns tend to rotate through different specialties. They may have an interest in obstetrics or may find it the most boring thing in the world.

Resident – Often referred to as RMO, or in some states as SHO, a resident is a year or two above an intern. These doctors are generally a bit more confident with basic patient care and are starting to develop an interest towards a certain specialty (including general practice or obstetrics). Many residents will have to complete 6 months of obstetric training on their way to general practice or another specialty. Residents are often relied on in public hospitals to do initial basic assessments on pregnant patients, and they are the most common staff who repair vaginal tears after birth in a lot of public hospitals.

Registrar – Is often in formal training to become a specialist obstetrician. In Australia, current registrar training to become a specialist is 6 years after acceptance into a program. For this reason, there is quite a bit of variation in experience between registrars, depending on how long they have been in training. In Australian public hospitals, most caesareans, vacuum and forceps deliveries are performed by registrars.

Career medical officer – Or CMO. These are doctors who have not formally trained to be either a GP or specialist obstetrician but have continued to work in public hospitals, often for many, many years. CMOs can often have a similar amount of experience to some obstetricians, especially with procedural skills, but have never sat formal examinations or met the training requirements to become a specialist.

Support persons

This is potentially the most important help you can have. A professional pregnancy support person is often referred to as a doula. The most common (non-professional) people in the room during labour are partners, mothers, mothers-in-law, sisters, friends, fathers, brothers, etc.

It is often suggested that you limit in-labour support people to two at a time. Having some people available to take relief shifts may also be useful. Common tasks for the support person may include massages, fetching drinks and snacks, putting down towels . . . But the most important job is just being there. The physical presence of a loved one during labour provides solidarity and motivation for the labouring woman. Sometimes, they may even be able to stand in as an advocate for plans made during the labour if the woman is exhausted, in distress or otherwise not able to speak for herself.

Home birth

Women have been giving birth for thousands of years. So why is it that now they need a doctor and a hospital to do it?

This is an argument that is often used against the 'interventional' trend in modern birth. It is true that as birth has become something that is more commonly done in a hospital, it has become more common for women to use medication for pain relief, or to undergo assisted births such as caesarean or vacuum delivery.

The counter-argument is that for thousands of years people accepted that it was not unusual to lose babies or mothers in childbirth. There is also little data to compare rates of bladder and bowel incontinence suffered by women in the past, or emotional trauma carried from poor birth outcomes. In Australian hospitals, deaths related to childbirth are very rare. The odds of a woman dying as a result of having a baby are around 1 in 10,000. The risk of a baby dying near the due date is 1 in 1000. A lot of this is due to modern surveillance and the ability to intervene when needed. However, it is true that when you draw a line somewhere with an intervention to prevent a tragedy, you want to draw that line with a fairly safe margin. This means that a proportion of women will end up having an intervention done as a precaution, when it might have been okay without it.

There is a growing movement towards women birthing out of hospital, which in part hopes to reverse the trend of intervention. Many programs designed to assist women to give birth in low-intervention environments, including in their home, are now available. For the most part, the people involved in these models of care are experienced and motivated practitioners. If you plan to give birth outside of hospital, do your research and make sure that your practitioner is working within the safe realm of their expertise. I would also encourage all women birthing outside of the hospital to engage with the hospital system in some way and have a fall-back plan in place. Trapeze artists can make their body do amazing things, but most would still like the safety net underneath them, just in case.

The key is finding the right balance between making use of medical care and being able to have the opportunity to keep things as natural as you would like them to be.

FIRST TRIMESTER TESTS

BLOOD GROUP, COUNT AND ANTIBODY SCREENING

There are various blood tests that are important during pregnancy. A blood count tells if your body has enough of the cells floating around that carry oxygen. These are called red cells, and the thing inside them that is most important for carrying oxygen is called haemoglobin. During pregnancy, your body needs to make about a litre of extra blood to have enough going around to supply oxygen to the placenta and baby. As part of this, your body also starts retaining more fluid to give the red cells something to float in. Sometimes you can make antibodies against foreign blood cells. Your baby may have a different blood type to you (like the father) and we screen to make sure your body's immune system is not reacting to this.

SCREENING FOR INFECTIONS AND IMMUNITY

Hepatitis, syphilis, HIV and rubella (German measles) are screened for in every pregnancy, so don't be offended when your doctor wants to order these tests. Based on your particular health history, the doctor may also order additional tests, such as serology for genital herpes, or checks for other bugs if you spend a lot of time with animals or small children. The reason for these checks is to look for viruses that may have an effect on your baby, either in relation to birth defects, or cross-infection during birth. Being forewarned in these circumstances can help to improve the outcome for your baby.

PAP SMEAR

This can be done in the first trimester but may be omitted due to the possibility of blood spotting after a pap smear, which can be alarming. If you are overdue for a pap smear, it is probably worth doing early in the pregnancy, but can often be safely left until 6 weeks after the baby is out if you are reasonably up to date. If you have recently had an abnormal pap smear, then it is important to have a discussion with an obstetrician about how this needs to be monitored during and after your pregnancy. Australian cervical cancer screening now involves testing for HPV DNA (the virus involved in abnormal pap smears) and is only required every 5 years.

ULTRASOUND

There are some women who choose to go through their entire pregnancy without having an ultrasound. While I respect the opinions of couples when it comes to this, it is recommended that all pregnant women have at least one ultrasound in the middle of the pregnancy, to know how many babies they are carrying, and to make sure the placenta is not blocking the way.

In the first trimester, there are a few reasons that an ultrasound may be suggested – to date the pregnancy, and to screen for early major birth defects and chromosomal disorders such as trisomy 21 (Down syndrome).

There are some additional reasons that an early ultrasound may be recommended by your doctor. These include any risk factors for ectopic pregnancy (see page 52), where an early pregnancy implants outside of the uterus. If undetected, this can be life-threatening, and in many women it can damage or even rupture a Fallopian tube. If detected early, it can often be managed without the need for surgery.

Dating

Dating of the pregnancy may not be necessary if you have a clockwork menstrual cycle and you are sure of your period dates. The dating scan can lead to confusion when it does not quite match up with your period dates. As a general principle, if your dates are within 5 days of an early ultrasound date, you can stick with them. Because the most consistent part of a woman's menstrual cycle is from ovulation to getting a period (14 days), women with longer cycles will actually be a bit earlier in the pregnancy using their first period date compared with women with shorter cycles. To naturally date a pregnancy, it is sometimes suggested that you subtract a number of days from your due date if your cycle is more than 28 days, or add a number of days to your due date if your cycle is shorter than 28 days. The most accurate time to date a pregnancy by ultrasound is between 8–10 weeks. At this stage, a heartbeat is clearly visible and there is not too much variation in size. At the end of a pregnancy, a healthy baby can vary from 2.5–5 kg (6–11 pounds), all of which can be perfectly normal for that particular couple. This variation in size begins after the first trimester, so dating a pregnancy after this time is notoriously inaccurate.

Be aware that it may not be possible to see a heartbeat until after 6 weeks of pregnancy. Even then, an internal ultrasound may be necessary to detect this. Most viable pregnancies should be visible with an ultrasound on your abdomen by 8 weeks' gestation – especially if you have a very full bladder. They are not just playing a joke on you by making you drink that litre of water before pushing on your bladder. The water in your bladder pushes the uterus up out of the pelvis and also provides a clear 'window' for the ultrasound waves to be reflected back to the probe. Keeping that bladder full for your dating scan will reduce the likelihood of the ultrasound technician having to use the internal probe (often referred to as 'the wand').

If the baby is not at the size you were expecting, don't be too worried until you see your doctor. There can often be a harmless reason and it may mean you ovulated late that cycle. Sometimes, it will be that the pregnancy has stopped developing at some point, which is referred to as a missed miscarriage. This can be a devastating experience (see pages 60–65 for more about miscarriage).

Screening

Some people feel that knowing whether or not they are carrying a child with a major chromosomal abnormality is important. This is a choice that you have to make for yourself, helped by good advice from your doctor. Ultrasound has been used for a number of years to measure the thickness at the back of the baby's neck – called the nuchal translucency – between 11–13 weeks. In conjunction with a blood test, this can give us an idea of the risk of your baby carrying an extra chromosome (called a trisomy) and having either Down syndrome (trisomy 21), Edwards syndrome (trisomy 18) or Patau syndrome (trisomy 13). More recently, these conditions can be detected by a blood test alone, called NIPT – non-invasive prenatal testing. However, as ultrasound technology improves, the 12-week scan has also been useful for picking up other major defects in the development of the baby's spine, brain, limbs or abdominal cavity. See pages 42–45 for more on chromosomal screening.

Is ultrasound safe for baby?

The technology uses high-frequency sound waves, which are a form of energy. In experimental studies using very high-powered ultrasound for extended periods of time (many hours, or even days), there have been temporary and reversible demonstrated changes in very particular tissue types shown in some animals. The implications of this are unknown in humans, using ultrasound at much lower power levels for only very brief durations, and not continually focusing on one tissue area. The risk, if any, of ultrasound is thought to be very, very small. Radiologists refer to this safe respectful use of imaging technology as the ALARA principle – as low as reasonably achievable. There are certain precautions we routinely take to minimise theoretical risks, such as avoiding high-power Doppler imaging on very early implantations or for prolonged periods of time near bone/fluid interfaces. Some people worry that ultrasound may be uncomfortable for the baby due to the pressure, or the perception of the sound. There is no evidence that ultrasound causes any recognisable distress for the baby. There is certainly no doubt that over many decades the ultrasound has revolutionised pregnancy management for the better.

What I'm really thinking . . .

The 12-week ultrasound

I was very nervous and excited as I neared the 12-week ultrasound, particularly in my first pregnancy. It is such a wonderful experience getting to see your baby for the first time. The ultrasound technician pointed out different parts of the body, but really, it all just looked like a blob! Then, she turned up the sound on the machine and there it was – the magical heartbeat! I felt an enormous sense of relief and joy that there was actually a tiny being growing inside of me. Hearing that heartbeat for the first time was like a weight had been lifted off my shoulders: it was all I had been longing to hear for the past 2 months.

FETAL DEVELOPMENT TO 20 WEEKS

In my practice, I look with the ultrasound at every visit. When it comes to development of the baby, I think in terms of what I can show the couple on a screen. In weeks 3 and 4, when some women may have an inkling that they are pregnant, if we look with an ultrasound, there will be a small cyst on the ovary (the one you ovulated from) and the uterus may look a little larger.

5 weeks

It is possible to confirm that a pregnancy is in the right place because a very small bubble will be visible inside the womb. This is the gestational sac, which is the developing amniotic fluid and early placental tissue. Until later in the pregnancy, the size of this sac is all we can measure to estimate how far along the pregnancy has progressed.

6 weeks

The gestational sac will be a lot bigger. It will generally be possible to see a tiny jellybean-shaped dot within this bubble, which is called a fetal pole. At this stage, the little jellybean is only a few mm long.

8 weeks

It should now be possible to see a flicker of a heartbeat. The rate of this heartbeat initially can be a little slow but should come up to a quite fast pace of 160 to 170 beats per minute (bpm) sometime during the next couple of weeks. The little jellybean may now even have visible limb buds, which look like stumpy little teddy-bear arms and legs. Sometimes, you can even see that baby still has a 'tail', as the rest of the baby catches up with the developing spine. It may be a little early to see any movement, but the bubble of fluid in the womb should be quite prominent.

10 weeks

The heartbeat should be easy to see. It will be possible to clearly see which end is the baby's head and which is the bottom. The little limbs will be starting to look like proper arms and legs. If you are lucky, you should be able to catch some movements of the baby, which often look like little jumps from the hips. But don't be too concerned if you don't see your baby move, as they can often sleep for long periods.

12 weeks

This is the most common time for women to have an ultrasound during the first trimester. By 12 weeks, the fetus is very obviously a baby. The bones are beginning to fill with calcium and, on ultrasound, begin to look like a little skeleton. The shape of the forehead and nose will be apparent. The spine and limb bones become obvious and the heartbeat is not just a flicker, but a proper beating heart. It will often be possible to actually hear the heartbeat by 12 weeks, using a Doppler ultrasound. Movements are common, and you may see the baby wave its hand, or arch its back. All of the major organ systems are formed, but are very tiny so are not able to be properly examined in detail. This is why we wait until closer to 20 weeks to have another look at all the organs.

16 weeks

A few weeks into the second trimester, most women will be able to feel their 'bump' above the pelvis and below the belly button, but may not yet be feeling movements. Baby weighs about 250 g and will be starting to get too big to fit on the ultrasound screen all at once. We are able to make out fine detail, such as fingers and toes. It may even be possible to have a reasonable guess about gender.

20 weeks

By now, all the organs are clearly visible on ultrasound, which is why we are able to check for anything untoward with development in the 'morphology ultrasound' (see page 80). From 20 weeks, it becomes possible to get a clear glimpse of the baby's face, with detail like the cheeks and lips becoming more apparent. The baby's gender is usually obvious, too, so make sure you tell the ultrasound technician if you don't want to know the sex of your baby.

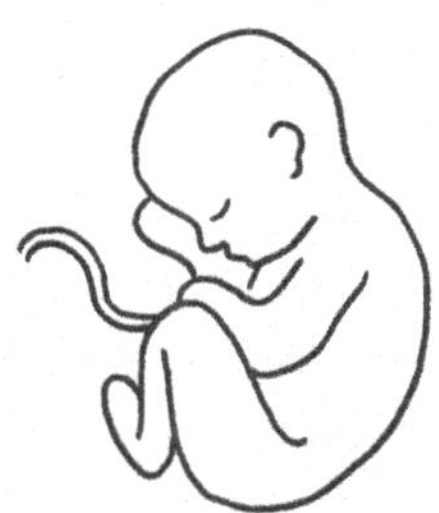

CHROMOSOMAL SCREENING – NUCHAL, NIPT AND INVASIVE TESTING

This area of testing has evolved rapidly in the past two decades. Chromosomal screening is now something that the majority of pregnant couples consider routine.

A chromosome is basically a big bundle of DNA, the stuff that carries our genes and makes us each as unique as we are. Inside every cell of our body is all of the genetic information, tightly organised into these chromosomes, of which most of us have 46. The only cells in our body that do not have 46 chromosomes are the ones we specifically use for making a baby. These are the sex cells, or gametes, and they are only supposed to have half of our chromosomes, 23. These are the sperm in men, and the ovum in women. When sperm are made, or ovum are getting ready to ovulate, they undergo a final molecular dance, in which a cell with all of our DNA is split into two, with half given to each gamete. Sometimes, this doesn't quite happen properly, and gametes with the wrong number of chromosomes are made.

For men, who make tens of thousands of sperm every day, producing a proportion of irregular sperm is considered normal. The age of the male partner does not seem to have as significant an impact as the woman on chromosome numbers for the baby. It is possible that the sperm with the bad chromosome combinations don't swim as well and can't fertilise the egg.

For women, each ovulation (once a month for most women) only releases one egg (but sometimes more, which is one way that twins occur). If that egg has an incorrect number of chromosomes, it is more of a problem for making a baby. This becomes more common with age in women, because all the eggs are present from the time a woman is born. 'Old' eggs don't seem to split their chromosomes as easily, and having the wrong number is more common.

When an egg is fertilised by a sperm, the chromosomes mix together: 23 from each parent usually makes an even 46 for the new baby. Out of the 23 pairs of chromosomes, there are some that are more vital than others to making a baby. Think of the chromosomes like the pages of an instruction manual for making a piece of flat-packed furniture – if you were reading the instructions and the last page with the warranty was missing, you could get by pretty well. If it was the page in the middle, which told you where to put those seven long screws and 22 short screws and that other thing with no name . . . you are probably going to struggle a bit more.

Most of the time, if the balance of chromosomes is wrong, the developing embryo realises it doesn't have all the instructions and the whole thing stops. This usually happens in the first 6 to 8 weeks and is the reason for a lot of miscarriages.

There are some combinations of chromosomes that aren't as readily recognised as challenging for the embryo, and it can develop into a more mature fetus without any obvious concerns. The most common combinations that allow an embryo to develop into the second trimester are the ones we screen for at the end of the first trimester. The chromosomes involved are numbered 13, 18 and 21. In addition, the sex chromosomes (X and Y) can also have uneven combinations. Some of the early pregnancy chromosomal tests will also screen for this.

Nuchal translucency

This test involves an ultrasound at around 12 weeks to check the thickness at the back of the baby's neck. A blood test is also taken from the mother to check for two substances, PAPP-A and free beta-HCG. The numbers from this ultrasound and the blood test are combined with statistics related to the mother's age and the incidence of major trisomies, and the odds of abnormality are calculated.

If you are in your 40s, and you have a 1 in 50 risk of having a baby with a chromosomal disability, a test result giving new odds of 1:700 is going to be pretty great news. This same result might sound terrifying to a woman in her early 20s, as her risk before the test was around 1:1400. It is still very unlikely that her baby has a syndrome, but to her mind, the risk just doubled.

NIPT

Non-invasive prenatal testing (NIPT) is a blood test for the mother that can detect tiny fragments of DNA from the baby floating around in the mother's bloodstream, called free fetal DNA.

This test can be performed from around 10 weeks onwards, and results are usually back within a week. Unlike nuchal translucency, the results are not affected as much by the age of the mother and they are not given as 'odds' but simply reported as low risk or high risk by the pathologist. For some labs, a 'low risk' result can be as low as 1:10 000, which most couples find reassuring.

Keep in mind that these results are currently limited to chromosomes 13, 18, 21, X, Y and some small partial chromosomal duplications or deletions.

It is also possible to be told the gender from this test, if you would like to know.

Who can have the test?

Anyone can have the NIPT test. If you are over 35, or you or your doctor would like to investigate further after the results of the 12-week ultrasound and scan, this may be an option for you.

What does it involve?

It involves a blood test anytime from week 10 onwards. The results are usually back within a week. If this result is low risk, few people would consider amniocentesis. If the result is high risk it would be likely that it is recommended to have amniocentesis to confirm the result before acting on it. Amniocentesis is a more invasive form of testing but it provides more accurate results. However, it is not a routine test and would only be undertaken if your doctor feels there is a need for further testing.

A modern-day dilemma of the NIPT test is that it can tell you the gender of the baby from as early as 10 weeks. Before this, most couples would have to wait for their second trimester ultrasound, which happens around 20 weeks, to know the gender. Don't worry: if you want to keep the gender a surprise (which is very common) you can choose for this result to be hidden from the lab report. If you do change your mind down the track, most laboratories will reveal the gender on request later.

Invasive prenatal testing

If any of the above screening tests return a positive result, confirming the condition requires a diagnostic test.

This is a test where a needle is inserted into the uterus through the skin of the abdomen, and some fluid is taken out of the sac around the baby (amniocentesis) or a small biopsy of placenta is collected (chorionic villus sampling or CVS). Screening for chromosomal problems is only one of the reasons these tests might be carried out, but it is the most common reason.

By taking a sample of fluid or tissue from around the baby and directly checking for chromosomal problems, you can be almost certain of the result. The biggest drawback of these tests has always been that they are invasive and hence carry a risk of complication, including a chance of causing a miscarriage of between 1 in 100 to 1 in 200, depending on the type of test.

What I'm really thinking . . .

The NIPT test

I didn't have the NIPT test with my first pregnancy, but decided that I wanted to do it with my second. It felt a little like doing a pregnancy test – a combination of excitement but also some anxiety, this time surrounding the health and wellbeing of my baby. In the end, I found that the test helped me to feel a lot less worried, because even if the results did indicate an abnormality, my husband and I could plan and prepare. And being as impatient as I am, I ticked the box to find out the gender of our baby – a perk of having the NIPT!

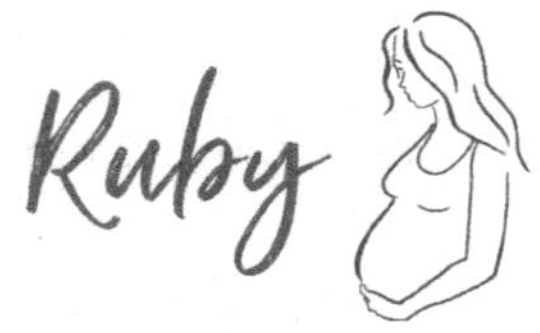

SYMPTOMS AND SIDE EFFECTS

Everyone has different experiences in the first trimester: some women breeze through without a twinge while others suffer from nausea and vomiting, tender breasts and/or low energy levels. These early symptoms may even be the first sign of pregnancy for you. Below is a list of the most common symptoms and side effects you may experience in the first few months of pregnancy.

MORNING SICKNESS

Morning sickness may be your first sign of pregnancy. From around week 6, you may start to feel nauseous or vomit, both of which are very common in early pregnancy. In fact, around half of pregnant women experience nausea or vomiting to some degree during the first trimester.

It is important to remember that morning sickness doesn't harm you or your baby. However, morning sickness that is severe and results in weight loss and dehydration may cause issues, and you should seek advice from your doctor (see page 48).

Medication is usually the last resort when it comes to treating nausea and vomiting during pregnancy. The two most widely used medications for women who suffer from moderate to severe nausea and vomiting are metoclopramide and ondansetron. Metoclopramide has recently become a category A medication, meaning it is safe to use while pregnant and has no known side effects in an unborn baby, while ondansetron is a category B medication, indicating that there are not enough adequate studies and research done in pregnant women.

If you experience vomiting and nausea that commences after week 9, it is a good idea to speak with your midwife or doctor to exclude other causes, such as illness or infection.

Tips for dealing with nausea:

- Eat small meals frequently.
- Snack on plain foods such as dry crackers or biscuits between meals. Keep crackers within arms' reach for when you first wake and feel nauseous or if you wake in the middle of the night.
- Avoid spicy or rich foods.
- Drink plenty of water to stay hydrated.
- Ginger may assist in easing nausea. You can safely take ginger tablets and drink ginger tea.
- Get plenty of rest.
- Changing to a multivitamin without iron may be beneficial for some women in managing nausea and vomiting, particularly during the first few weeks until the symptoms subside.

What I'm really thinking . . .

Morning sickness

My nausea in the first 12 weeks was debilitating and had a real impact on my excitement about being pregnant. All I wanted to do was hide away at home, with a bucket next to my bed, sipping on ginger tea or sucking on ice blocks. Cooking was just awful, with every smell making me feel more nauseous. I kept reminding myself that the nausea was a good thing – it meant my pregnancy hormone levels were high, which in turn meant it was highly likely my pregnancy was going to continue.

Nausea in my second pregnancy was even more dreadful: running after a toddler while wanting to throw up is never a good time! This is where help from my partner, family and friends was essential. Rest helped to ease the nausea, as did snacking on dry crackers. It was such a relief when the nausea eventually passed at the start of the second trimester.

David

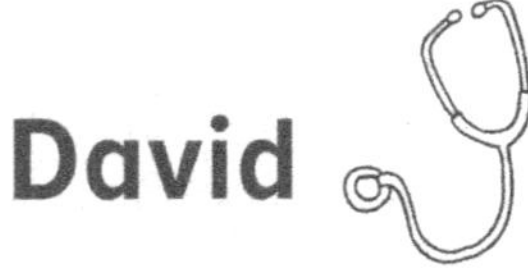

HYPEREMESIS GRAVIDARUM

Hyperemesis gravidarum is the medical term for severe nausea and vomiting in pregnancy. It can begin as early as the first 4–6 weeks and can cause weight loss and dehydration. It requires medical attention and, sometimes, hospitalisation.

Nausea and vomiting in pregnancy is considered a problem when any of the following start happening:

- You become dehydrated.
- You lose weight.
- You show signs of nutritional deficiency or anaemia.
- It is having a significant impact on your mental health and wellbeing.

Women with hyperemesis are among the most distressed patients I come across. In severe cases, this can be truly debilitating. Many women require anti-nausea medication and multiple admissions to hospital during the first trimester for intravenous fluid rehydration. It is uncommon, but possible, to become so malnourished and unwell from this condition that it can cause organ dysfunction in the mother and lead to extreme measures, such as intensive care unit admission and use of intravenous nutrition.

There are a number of medications that doctors can prescribe for hyperemesis. Some of these have a well-established safety record, while some are not known to cause problems but do not have an established safety record, so must be used with caution. Last-line medications have a small potential for harm or side effects.

In addition to lifestyle and dietary measures, doctors will usually gradually build on the medications until the nausea is controlled.

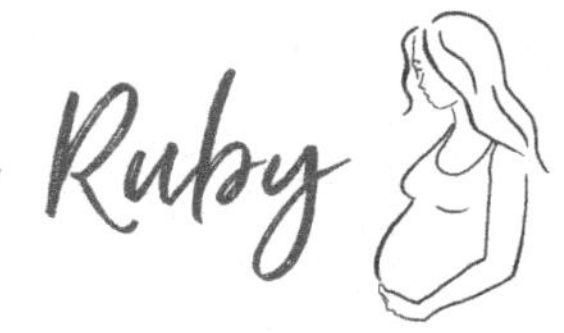

BLEEDING

Light bleeding or spotting is common in early pregnancy. Though distressing, it is not necessarily a sign of an impending miscarriage. If you have light spotting around 8 days after ovulation, it may be what is known as endometrial implantation bleeding. If you have noticed some spotting, you may find that using a panty liner is beneficial as it will allow you to keep an eye on the consistency and quantity of blood. If you notice bleeding that is heavy or accompanied by cramping, seek medical advice from either your doctor or midwife.

BREAST CHANGES

Be prepared for many breast changes throughout your pregnancy, especially as you near birth and prepare to produce milk. Swollen and tender breasts are normal in the first trimester, and may be similar to what you experience when your period is due. You may notice the veins on your breasts become more visible, and your nipples darken in colour and feel sensitive to touch. A supportive bra with no underwire may help to alleviate tenderness.

CRAMPING AND PAIN

Mild cramping in early pregnancy is common. Cramping or stomach aches and pains are usually due to ligaments stretching around your growing uterus. Back pain is also a common complaint, as your stomach begins to grow, putting increased pressure on your lower back. If cramping or stomach pain is severe, or accompanied by bleeding, vomiting, fever or urinary tract symptoms, or if you are worried, speak with your midwife or doctor to ensure there aren't any other underlying issues.

BLOATING

Many women experience bloating in the first trimester due to the hormone progesterone, which causes your digestive system to slow down and, in turn, makes you feel bloated and uncomfortable.

CONSTIPATION

Constipation is a common complaint during pregnancy, but one that women tend not to discuss. Constipation can be due to the increase in progesterone slowing down the digestive system, and the surge of blood volume and fluid being retained in the bowel. There are also other causes of constipation, including the pressure of your expanding uterus on the intestines; however, this is more the case in the second and third trimester.

To treat constipation, first increase your dietary fibre by eating more fruit, vegetables and whole grains. Try adding psyllium husk to smoothies, porridge and baked goods (but make sure you increase your fluid intake too). If there are no improvements, osmotic laxatives such as lactulose and macrogol are safe to use. These draw fluid to the bowel to encourage a soft stool, rather than causing cramping and contractions in the bowel, which are counterproductive. These laxatives are commonly used in pregnancy, and also for mothers who suffer from constipation after birth. Another option, which you may prefer to leave as your last resort, is glycerol suppositories. These are very safe, gentle and fast-acting.

VAGINAL DISCHARGE

You may have noticed an increase in vaginal discharge since discovering you are pregnant. This happens due to the forming of the mucus plug around the opening of your cervix, which protects your baby during pregnancy. There is no need to worry about this common symptom. Vaginal discharge can increase in the third trimester, or as you near your due date. This is normal. You may decide to wear a panty liner to feel a little more comfortable.

If you have a burning sensation and pain during urination, this may be a sign of a urinary tract infection. Urinary tract infections need be treated so make your doctor aware if you experience any of these symptoms while pregnant.

FATIGUE

A common complaint from women in the first trimester is feeling fatigued. If this is you, the good news is there is nothing to worry about except focusing on getting plenty of rest. The bad news is that fatigue can continue throughout your entire pregnancy. However, you may start to feel as though you have more energy as you enter the second trimester. In the meantime, taking time to relax (particularly if you have a stressful or physical job), keeping hydrated, eating well and engaging in low-impact exercise daily will all help.

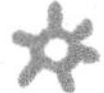

ANNOUNCING YOUR PREGNANCY

When it comes to sharing the news of your pregnancy with family and friends, decide with your partner when is the best time for you. This may be before or after the 12-week scan. You may choose to announce it through social media, or you may prefer to have immediate family members together to share the exciting news. You might send a photo or even plan a dinner and tell all your loved ones at the same time. (When I told my parents about my pregnancy, I was so nervous that I spent the whole weekend with them before I got the nerve to tell them – just as we were leaving!)

It can be difficult sharing your announcement with a friend or loved one who has miscarried or is having trouble conceiving. Be mindful that they may want to hear the news from you, rather than on social media or through a friend. Take the time to sit down with them and show them that you care about how they feel. Accept that it will be bittersweet for them. They will be delighted to hear your news, but they may also feel a sense of sadness, or even resentment, too. For many of us who have miscarried or have fertility issues, it can be difficult hearing the news of someone else's pregnancy. Attending baby showers and children's birthday parties can also be upsetting, so don't be offended if that friend doesn't attend.

David

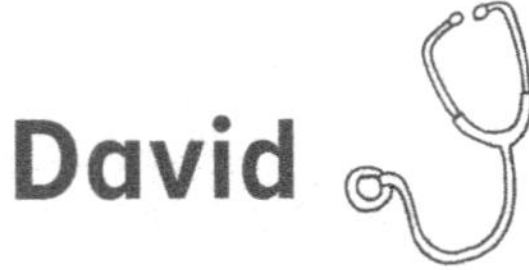

ECTOPIC PREGNANCY

The word ectopic, in medical terms, means something growing where it shouldn't be. A pregnancy should grow in the middle of the uterus. If it happens anywhere else in the body, it is called ectopic. Fortunately, this doesn't happen all that often. Around 1 in 200 pregnancies is ectopic.

In the vast majority of cases, if a pregnancy is not in the right place, it is in a fallopian tube. This is the passage from the ovary into the womb.

Most women are born with two fallopian tubes, one on each side. They are 8–10 cm long and less than 1 cm wide. Conception occurs in the fallopian tubes, where the sperm fertilises a newly ovulated egg. As the fertilised egg travels down the tube, it is helped by fine hair-like structures called cilia, which sweep the fertilised egg in the right direction into the womb. This can take close to a week.

Sometimes, the embryo doesn't make it all the way to the end of the tube before it starts to implant. This can then result in a fallopian tube ectopic pregnancy. A lot of the time, this just happens because of bad luck. However, it is more likely to happen if there has been damage to the tubes as a result of pelvic infections, pelvic surgery or previous ectopic pregnancies.

A small number of ectopic pregnancies do not occur in the fallopian tube; other places include the muscular corner of the womb (cornua), the cervix, or inside the abdominal cavity on the surface of the pelvis, ovary or even the bowel.

The most common way that a pregnancy is found to be ectopic is because it has caused pain from stretching the tube. Occasionally, it can start to bleed, which can then become dangerous, and even life-threatening.

How is an ectopic pregnancy treated?

Unfortunately, there is no way to save an ectopic pregnancy and put it in the right place. This means that ectopic pregnancies are a form of miscarriage. It is a difficult situation, as often the woman has only recently discovered she is pregnant, only to then have to come to terms with this loss. On top of that, she is told she has a potentially life-threatening condition that requires urgent treatment.

Sometimes, an ectopic pregnancy will resolve naturally, called a tubal miscarriage. But because ectopic pregnancy has the potential to cause severe internal bleeding, most doctors will not adopt a 'wait and see' approach, beyond being sure that they have made the correct diagnosis. The options are surgery, or medication to stop the pregnancy before it goes any further.

Most surgery for ectopic pregnancies is done by keyhole laparoscopy. Depending on whether the ectopic pregnancy has begun to damage the tube, or has started bleeding, there is a high chance that the patient may lose one of her fallopian tubes in surgery, which obviously adds another layer of grief. In certain circumstances, though, the tube can be opened to remove the ectopic without removing the tube.

Medication can be used if the ectopic pregnancy is diagnosed early, as long as there is no sign of internal bleeding or significant pain. The most common drug used to treat ectopic pregnancy in Australia is methotrexate, which stops cells being able to reproduce. The dose only rarely causes side effects. It is recommended that women who have this drug should not conceive a new pregnancy for up to 3 months, to be sure the drug is completely out of their system.

Women who have had an ectopic pregnancy should be aware that they are at an increased risk of it happening again. This is especially true if the damaged tube is left behind. Women who lose one tube still have quite good fertility outcomes though. If one tube is gone, fertility is not reduced by 50 per cent (as you might imagine) but only 15–20 per cent compared to women with both tubes. This is because a single healthy tube can pick up eggs from both ovaries. I encourage women who have suffered an ectopic pregnancy to be cautiously optimistic for a future pregnancy, but also to make sure that they have an early ultrasound and medical review to ensure that history does not repeat itself.

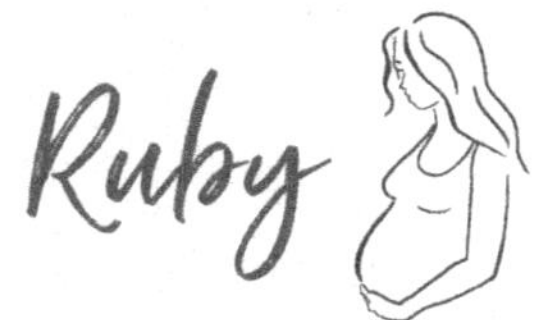

EXPECTING TWINS

Since I have not had the pleasure of birthing twins, I have enlisted the help of friends and family members to share their experience and advice for women who are expecting twins:

- Pregnancy symptoms can occur earlier and may be more intense when carrying twins, because your pregnancy hormone levels will be higher. Nausea, heartburn and fatigue can all be more severe in twin pregnancy.
- Get in touch with support services and classes specifically for parents expecting twins or multiples, such as the Australian Multiple Birth Association (AMBA).
- Consider joining Facebook groups for women expecting twins. Read articles or blogs written by mothers of twins to gain an insight into what it is really like.
- Expect to gain more weight than you would with a single pregnancy – you are carrying two babies, two placentas and a lot of extra fluid.
- There will be even more pressure down below, so do those pelvic floor exercises! Starting these early will ensure you keep a strong pelvic floor and reduce the likelihood of prolapse.
- Being pregnant with twins is more demanding physically and mentally, so if you are exhausted, don't push yourself – give yourself plenty of time to take a break and rest. Remember you are carrying two babies!
- Write a checklist of all the items you will need: a double pram, two bassinets, two cots, etc. That said, just because you're having twins doesn't mean you need to buy two of everything.
- People are curious about twin pregnancies, so do be prepared for questions, but know that you have a right to privacy – you do not have to discuss anything you don't feel comfortable with.

- Be prepared that it may be challenging towards the end of your pregnancy as the heaviness makes it difficult to keep active. You may find that light walking or swimming are the only exercises you feel like doing.
- As the weeks go by, you might be preparing for your babies to come early and need to get things in order a little sooner than women with a single pregnancy.
- It's a good idea to discuss alterations that may need to be made to your job role to make your pregnancy easier in the later months.
- You may want to discuss options for feeding with your doctor or midwife. Some women choose to pump breastmilk and feed their babies with a bottle, which allows partners or family members to assist at feeding times. Some women choose to breastfeed both babies (yes, this is possible), and others prefer to use formula.
- If your babies are born prematurely, they may have to stay in hospital for a number of days or weeks until they reach a certain weight and are given the all-clear to go home. If you are discharged from hospital during this time, take the opportunity to get plenty of sleep and allow your body to recover and rest before your babies come home.
- It is safest for your babies to sleep in separate cots, although many twins in the early weeks sleep 'top and tail' in the same cot.

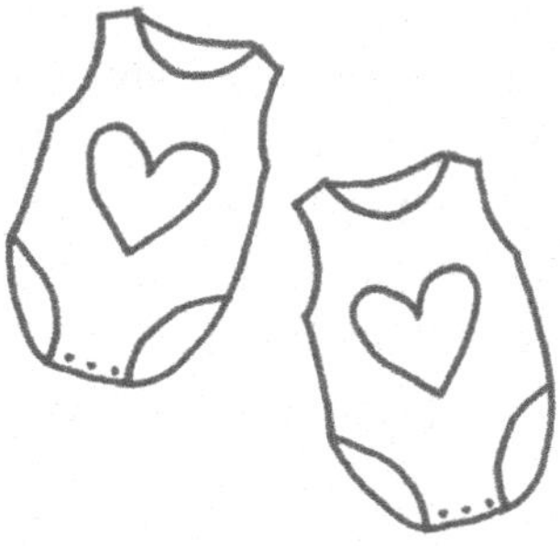

What I'm really thinking:

Expecting twins

I suppose a lot of the questions are the same as any first-time mum: *Will my belly and my boobs ever be the same? Will I end up with stretch marks like a patchwork quilt? What on earth is the birth going to be like?* I do recall feeling lucky and proud amidst the concern for the practicalities. There seems to be an extra frisson of excitement when people find out that you are having twins (and many more questions!).

From the start, I felt the need to arm myself with information. I sought out mums of twins, attended multiple-birth antenatal classes and joined twin-birth clubs to try to gain some insight into my future. I found this to be really helpful.

At the time, I didn't completely understand what having a 'high-risk' pregnancy really meant and felt mild annoyance that I wouldn't be able to give birth at the local hospital. But later on, I was enormously grateful to have been monitored so diligently and to have given birth in a hospital with access to high-tech medical facilities.

Rosie, mum of fraternal twins

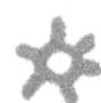

DEALING WITH UNSOLICITED ADVICE

People love to give unsolicited advice – and it doesn't stop at the end of pregnancy; it just moves on to unwanted parenting advice! While most of it is well-intentioned, it can also be quite confronting. Whether it be delivered by your mum, mother-in-law, friends, family members, midwives, even the person who serves you at the local supermarket, you will no doubt at some point experience unwelcome comments on the progress of your pregnancy.

It is best to take advice from someone knowledgeable and who you feel you can trust. This could be your own mum, your best friend, your midwife or your doctor. It is also important to trust your instincts. You of all people know your body, and trusting in yourself may help you to make the best decisions for you and your baby. People will offer advice on everything: breastfeeding, birthing options, avoiding weight gain, having a C-section . . . the list goes on.

Here are a few tips to help you navigate unwanted comments:

- Plan. Have a few go-to responses when it comes to questions such as 'Are you going to have a natural birth?' or 'Are you going to breastfeed?'. Come up with a few generic answers, such as 'I haven't yet decided' or 'I haven't thought that far ahead'.
- Ask yourself, 'Is this advice useful for me?'
- Use humour to deflect unwanted comments or suggestions.
- Be honest. If a comment is truly offensive or upsetting, let the person know how you feel, especially if they are someone you have a lot of contact with.

Having a baby after 35

As you reach your 30s, you hear about how a woman's fertility decreases and the risks during pregnancy increase. Indeed, in medical terms, if you are a pregnant woman over 35, you are considered 'of advanced maternal age' and therefore classified as 'high risk'.

Yet, more and more women are now starting their families in their 30s, some even later. Many women may not feel ready to embark on motherhood in their 20s, or they don't meet the right partner until their 30s.

There are many upsides to having a baby later in life:

- Improved job security: gender equality in the workplace has given us the opportunity to study and work with a focus on building a career before starting a family.
- Improved financial stability.
- Broader life experience: you may have travelled, studied or worked overseas.

To put it in perspective: the average age of pregnant women giving birth in Australia is 30.1 years.

WORK AND CAREER

It doesn't matter what age you are when you decide to start a family, at some point you will question how it will affect your paid employment: *How might it affect my career? Will I miss out on a promotion because I am pregnant or a new mother? Will I be able to go back to work when I want to? Will I be able to study in the future to enhance my career prospects?*

More than any time in history, women are focused on remaining in the workforce while being mothers. I constantly reminded myself of this fact throughout my pregnancy – and that although adjustments need to be made once your baby comes along, there are options available to women who want to return to the workforce.

Here are a few tips I learned from my own experience:

- If you know when you will return to work, getting organised and planning ahead is very important.
- Be realistic – it is definitely a juggling act.
- Research childcare options and put your name down early.
- Ask family members and friends about how they coped with the transition back to work.
- Talk to your employer about different work arrangements available to you. By law, your employers are required to provide maternity leave and to make adjustments to your job role to enable you to return to work. If you feel that your employer is unsupportive, or you are experiencing discrimination in the workplace, discuss this with your employer or human resources department. Alternatively, you can discuss your entitlements and rights with the Fair Work Ombudsman.

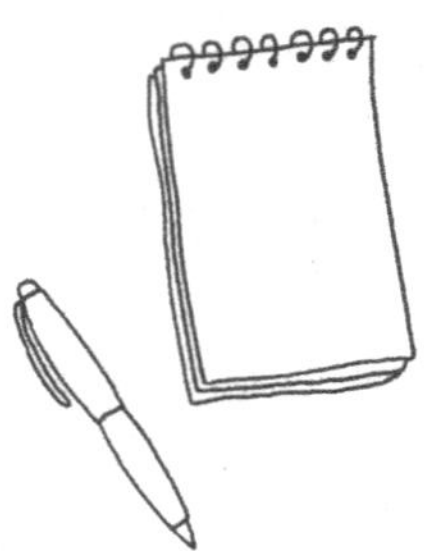

TELLING YOUR EMPLOYER YOU'RE PREGNANT

While there are laws in place to protect pregnant women, it can still be daunting sharing your pregnancy news with your employer. Most women wait until after the 12-week scan, although you may decide to tell your employer earlier, particularly if you are affected by early pregnancy symptoms such as hyperemesis.

Here are some things you may need to discuss with your current employer:

- Changes to your current role, such as limiting heavy lifting, chemical exposures or travel for the duration of your pregnancy.
- Attending appointments throughout your pregnancy.
- Maternity leave.
- Return-to-work entitlements and adjustments. You may be entitled to paid parental leave at your workplace. If you receive paid parental leave from the government, you will need to meet certain work requirements. Your partner should also confirm their leave entitlements with their own employer.

Budgeting for a baby

Taking steps to get your finances in order before baby arrives is a smart idea. It can alleviate any worries or stresses down the track when your focus will be on feeding and sleeping. Begin by researching the government's paid parental leave scheme, and finding out what your employer offers in regards to parental leave. Draw up a budget for the time you have off work. Now is a good time to review non-essential outgoings for things you may not necessarily need or use after your baby arrives e.g. membership to a gym near your work or a subscription to a magazine you no longer read, etc.

David

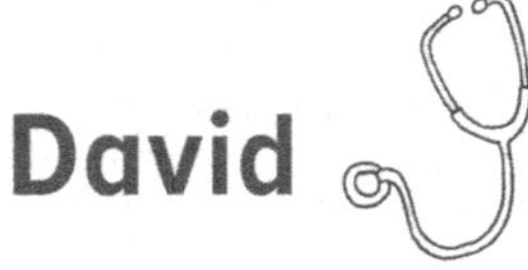

MISCARRIAGE

For a lot of women, the possibility of miscarriage is constantly in the back of their minds during the early months of pregnancy.

Miscarriage is a general term for a pregnancy that doesn't continue past 20 weeks, though most happen in the first trimester, largely by about 8 weeks. A miscarriage early in the second trimester is sometimes called a 'late miscarriage'. In Australia, a pregnancy loss after 20 weeks legally requires birth and death certificates, and is referred to as a stillbirth.

When you use a home pregnancy kit, it detects part of a hormone in your urine called human chorionic gonadotrophin, or more easily pronounced as hCG. This is a hormone produced by the developing placental tissue after an embryo begins to stick to the uterine wall. Some of the newer home pregnancy kits can detect very low levels of this, which can even show a positive result before your period is due. This is a potential reason why very early miscarriages, or 'chemical pregnancies', are becoming more commonly recognised.

If you've ever had a very early miscarriage, you'll know that you experience the same intense loss that you would with a more developed pregnancy. Physically though, you may only experience a slightly late and perhaps heavier period. And it happens a lot more than most people realise.

The overall rate of miscarriage in the first trimester is around 1 in 6 pregnancies, though a lot of factors change these odds. Age is a big one. If you are in your 20s, your risk is about 1 in 10. If you are in your 40s, it is about 1 in 2. This is an inescapable biological reality that comes down to the age of the eggs in your ovaries, and the way the chromosomes split when you ovulate. There are some modifiable lifestyle factors as well, such as obesity and smoking. Some are inherent to the genetics and immune systems of the couple.

How do you know if a pregnancy has failed?

The physical signs of losing an early pregnancy are bleeding and cramping very similar to period pain. Often these symptoms may not occur until some weeks after a pregnancy stops developing. During this time the woman may not 'feel pregnant' due to the symptoms of pregnancy stopping, or they may not feel different at all. This is referred to by doctors as a missed miscarriage, because the pregnancy has failed but the body has not yet realised it.

To determine that a pregnancy has failed, generally either ultrasound and a blood test for hCG are used.

By ultrasound, a heartbeat should be easily visible by about 8 weeks from the last period. Often, without a heartbeat seen, if you or the doctor are concerned that the pregnancy is not continuing, a repeat ultrasound may be requested in 7–10 days to see if things are changing. This can be an anxious wait for couples.

The blood test for hCG can be used in this situation to help make it clear if a pregnancy is continuing or not. On average, with continuing pregnancies, the level on a blood test should double every two days. Occasionally, a pregnancy will still be continuing even if the level only rises a small amount. If the hCG level has not risen at all, or started to fall, and there is no visible heartbeat, the pregnancy is not successful.

Most maternity hospitals in Australia have special clinics to help women deal with pregnancy loss, often called an early pregnancy assessment unit, service or clinic (respectively EPAU, EPAS or EPAC). Most GPs can help with this initial stage of checking on early pregnancies as well.

Treatment of miscarriage

Not all miscarriages start with cramping and bleeding. With the sensitivity of modern ultrasound and blood tests, most miscarriages are diagnosed well before your body has a chance to react. In principle, if you keep waiting, things will usually happen. This is called the expectant approach to miscarriage.

If you want the help for things to happen quicker, the options are medication to help your body start the process, or a surgical procedure to empty the uterus.

- *Expectant management.* Also termed 'supported waiting'. In an early pregnancy, hormonal signals are sent between the ovary and the early pregnancy tissue in the womb. They support each other to continue progressing. When a pregnancy fails, it can be a number of weeks before these signals stop, and your body physically starts to miscarry. On average, the amount of pain and bleeding from a miscarriage will be heavier than a period, but should still be manageable at home if you are comfortable with this. Depending on how far along the pregnancy was, you may also pass tissue that looks different from a period. Understandably, a lot of women worry about seeing the fetus. In general, prior to 10 weeks gestation, the tissue that passes just looks like a small placenta, or thick, pale menstrual tissue. If the pregnancy progresses past 11 weeks gestation, the baby can become more obvious, and after 13 weeks, it is quite clearly formed. In rare cases, either during or following a miscarriage, bleeding can become excessive, requiring the woman to come to hospital for help to complete the miscarriage and manage any bleeding. When the bleeding stops, it is a good sign that everything has come away.
- *Medical management.* With this strategy, medication is given to help your body start the process of a natural miscarriage. Most Australian hospitals administer this medication and allow patients to go home to await events. The medication used is generally very safe, but can occasionally result in minor side effects, such as a mild fever. As with a natural miscarriage, occasionally the process may be drawn out, or bleeding may be excessive, requiring fall-back to a surgical approach.
- *Surgical management.* While the idea of a surgical procedure may not be a nice one for some people, it does provide definite closure. Emotionally, this can be easier for a lot of women, but physically, it does expose them to risk, however minor, from undergoing an operation. The procedure is done under anaesthetic, and usually takes less than 10 minutes. There is no cutting or stitching. An 8–10 mm wide, plastic suction tube is placed into the womb and the tissue is removed. Bleeding and cramping usually settle in less than a week. There is a small chance of pregnancy tissue being left behind or, very rarely, of introducing bacterial infection or causing damage to the uterus.

When is it safe to try again?

If your body lets you fall pregnant, it is safe and you are physically ready. Being emotionally ready is a different matter, and you should consider giving yourself time to grieve a pregnancy loss before a new one begins. It can also be easier if you have had a normal period cycle in between pregnancies, because it gives reassurance that your body has healed, and the certainty of your period dates will make knowing how far along you are in a new pregnancy much easier to tell.

While it is important to recognise and grieve a lost pregnancy, there is no value in dwelling on causes. Most miscarriages have nothing to do with anything the woman did, and are the result of a particular combination of egg and sperm. Most women will be successful the next try. Only occasionally does this become a recurrent issue.

Recurrent miscarriage

When a couple experience a string of miscarriages, this is often a prompt to go looking for causes. Most of the time, no cause for recurrent miscarriages is found. The testing can be very expensive, and some of the results can take many weeks.

While we know of a large number of medical conditions associated with miscarriage, very few of them have easy cures. Better management of long-term medical problems (such as thyroid problems or diabetes) can improve miscarriage odds. If a genetic cause is found, often this requires other means to be considered, such as IVF. There are some chromosomal combinations, called translocations, which can be carried by perfectly 'normal' people, but which cause the sperm or eggs to be genetically imbalanced.

There are a couple of identified causes that do have some remedies. One condition, called antiphospholipid syndrome, can respond to low-dose aspirin and/or a prescribed blood thinning injection.

More recent research is focusing on the immune system. It is thought that some women have an overactive immune system, which fights an embryo in the same way it might fight bacteria or a virus. While there is some promise using medications which dull the immune system, this is an area which needs more research.

Treatments to discuss with your doctor

Below are a few medications which have been studied in relation to pregnancy loss in the first trimester. The limited evidence for each treatment is for specific conditions only and may be harmful if used in the wrong instance. Take to your doctor about your own situation before taking any medication.

- Aspirin (oral blood thinner and anti-inflammatory).
- Heparin (injectable blood thinner).
- Progesterone (hormone medication, usually given as a cream or vaginal pessary and mainly studied in relation to IVF pregnancies).
- Metformin (a diabetes drug, which is mainly studied in relation to polycystic ovarian syndrome and miscarriage).
- Prednisone (steroid tablets, which can address irregularities with the immune system).
- High-dose folic acid (5 mg folate, which is more than a typical pregnancy multivitamin contains). This is strongly advised for diabetics and women with a history of pregnancies where the baby had a neural tube defect.

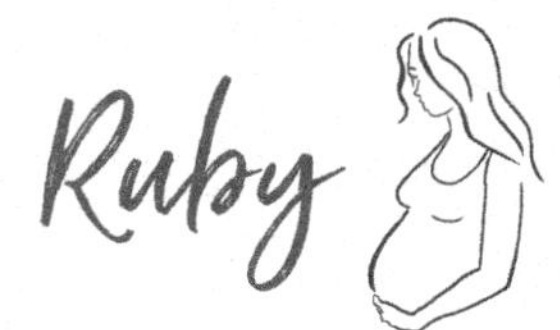

RECOVERING FROM MISCARRIAGE

It doesn't matter how far along you were, miscarriage can be devastating. Grief is grief, and most of us suffer in silence. Even though the doctor gives you the all-clear to start trying to conceive again, it is okay to grieve for the baby you have lost.

- Take time. Talk when you feel ready and to whom you feel most comfortable and supported by, whether that be your partner, friend, family member or a professional.
- There is no time-frame for recovery. Everyone deals with miscarriage in different ways emotionally and mentally. Let yourself grieve.
- Respect that your partner may also be grieving. Although they have not physically experienced a miscarriage, they are often just as emotionally affected, and you can find peace in knowing they understand what you are going through.
- Plant a tree. You might find that something symbolic of new life, such as planting a tree, can help ease the grief.
- If you need extra support and advice, seek professional help from a counsellor or psychologist. Speaking with professionals can be very beneficial as they are not emotionally attached to you and can help you address your fears and anxieties.

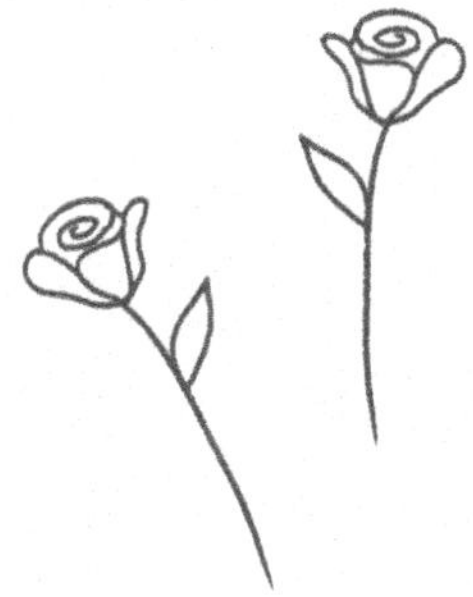

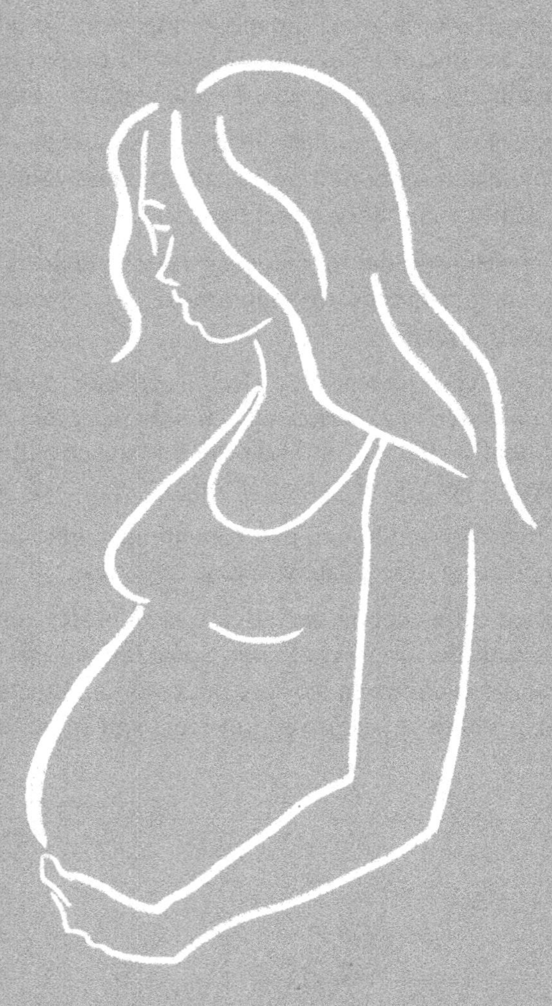

SECOND TRIMESTER

David

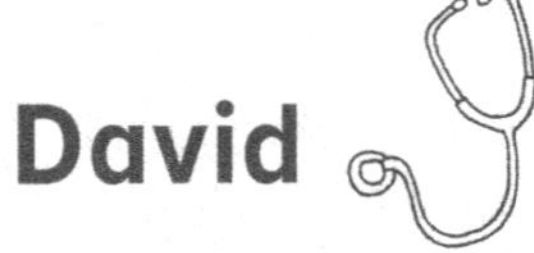

I call the second trimester the 'honeymoon period' because your body has hopefully settled in to a lot of the hormonal and physiological changes of pregnancy, such as nausea and fatigue, but your baby is still not big enough to put too much pressure on your pelvis and diaphragm.

As you enter the second trimester, your baby has functioning organs, nerves and muscles. Baby's skin is transparent, and the sex may be visible enough to see on a scan. The bones are beginning to harden, the digestive system is working, and the lungs are developing. Your baby can even begin to hear you – and it won't be long until you feel its first movements.

Ruby

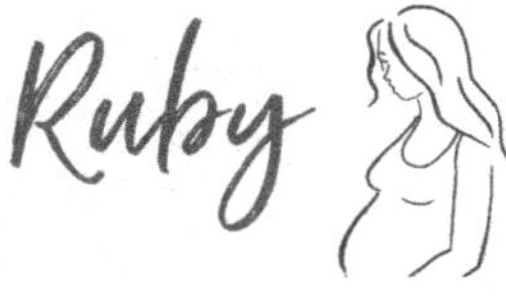

THE 'HONEYMOON PERIOD'

This is when you can breathe a sigh of relief after making it through the first trimester and start to enjoy the pregnancy. Usually, not too much happens medically speaking in the second trimester. Most doctors and midwives will advise a check-up at least every 4 weeks and at around 20 weeks an ultrasound is recommended to check that the baby is developing normally.

Towards the end of second trimester (26–28 weeks) some additional blood tests are recommended to check for anaemia (see page 88) and changes in sugar metabolism (gestational diabetes; see page 83).

The second trimester is a special time, as it is when you will start to feel those kicks and rolling movements in your growing belly. It's these moments that make all those pregnancy symptoms worth living with.

You look down and see a nice round bump that people no longer mistake as simply weight gain. The excitement and anticipation is heightening and it is all starting to feel very real. If you are lucky enough, you may start to feel a little more 'normal' as some of the pregnancy symptoms experienced in the first trimester begin to settle. If you are thinking about going on a little getaway (otherwise known as a 'babymoon'), this is the trimester to do it in; you're not yet waddling or feeling uncomfortable, making travelling a little easier (see page 111).

I have never had curves, and the second trimester was the best part of both my pregnancies because I finally got 'those' curves. I felt more relaxed knowing the results of the scans and, with some of those pregnancy symptoms easing, I could start to enjoy being pregnant. The second trimester was when I felt like exercising again (see page 94) and I also began to think about finishing work projects, knowing that it wouldn't be long until I would be on maternity leave.

Some things your partner can do:

- Give compliments! Your pregnant partner may be feeling self-conscious or anxious, so don't forget to give her honest compliments, and let her know she is doing a good job.
- Offer a foot massage or a back rub.
- Take charge of creating some special time – cook a meal, organise a date night or plan a babymoon.
- Attend antenatal or birthing classes.

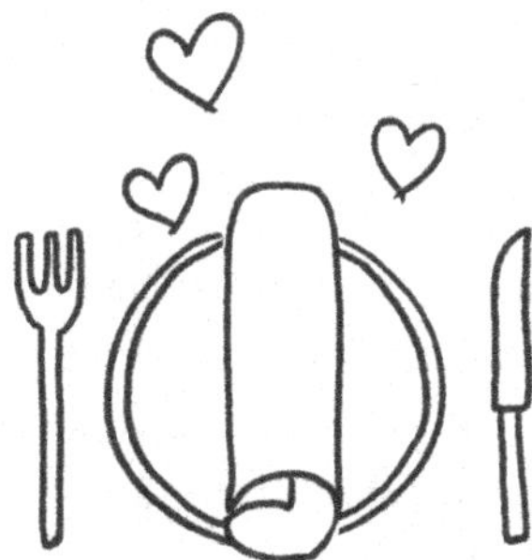

David

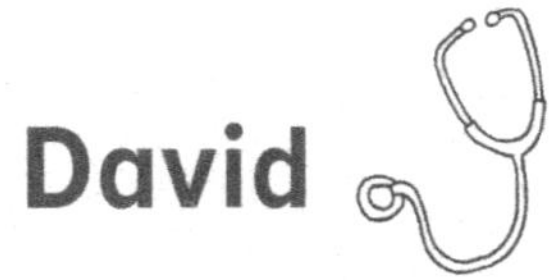

WHAT TO EXPECT AT CHECK-UPS

There are some basic checks that should be done every visit with your care provider. Your blood pressure should be taken. The baby's heartbeat should be heard (especially after 12 weeks). The doctor or midwife will want to feel your abdomen and check the size of your uterus. They may check your ankles for swelling or listen to your chest. As the baby gets bigger, they will be able to feel for position and how low, or 'engaged', the baby is. A lot of obstetricians will make routine use of ultrasound, which is much more reliable at confirming the position of the baby, and also allows additional information about the fluid around baby, flow through the umbilical cord, and growth.

Most pregnancy care providers in Australia make use of a hand-held pregnancy record, a card or a booklet which is given to the woman to keep with her. It contains a summary of all the relevant tests and health information which doctors and midwives like to know about. We recommend that pregnant women keep it with them at most times, particularly if away from home or their usual care provider, such as on holiday or work trips. If you have an unexpected concern which requires coming in to the hospital, it is useful for the staff to have a quick summary of all your care, especially in an emergency. These hand-held records are also a convenient way to keep track of check-ups with different care providers during a pregnancy. At every visit with your GP, midwife or obstetrician, they should write a summary of your check-up and any issues identified or concerns discussed. Below are the typical boxes you may see on your hand-held record for each check-up and what they mean.

Blood pressure (BP)

Written down as two numbers. This is the upper and lower limit of pressure in your arteries when your heart beats. The number refers to 'millimetres of mercury' and relates back to the old mercury column devices that doctors used and how high the column rose. These days, it is rare to see a mercury device, but the unit of measurement persists. Average blood pressure is around 120/80 mmHg (millimetres of mercury). In pregnancy, it can get much lower. As long as you don't get dizzy or faint, this is generally not a problem. High blood pressure can be, however (see page 135).

Fundal height (FH)

By about 16 weeks, it should be possible to feel the top of your uterus (fundus) just above the underwear line. By 20 weeks, this should be at around the level of your belly button. By 37 weeks, your uterus will be just under your ribs. Usually we measure the growth of the uterus with a tape measure from the fundus to the middle of the pubic bone. This is called the fundal height. Conveniently, the fundal height is, on average, 1 cm for every week along in the pregnancy. Variations up to 2 cm either way can be normal, but variation may be a trigger to suggest an ultrasound to check how the baby is growing. This measurement is influenced by a lot of other factors, such as your weight and body shape, how low the baby's head is or which way it is lying. The fundal height can also be very subjective between care providers and the way they measure you.

Fetal heart rate (FHR)

Hearing the baby's heart is one of the things most couples look forward to with their check-up. Most practitioners will use a Doppler, or, rarely, a Pinard stethoscope, which is like a long skinny trumpet. This allows a doctor or midwife to listen to the heart of the baby directly, but the woman herself cannot hear. These days, Pinards are mainly a curiosity or museum ornament, but can be useful for couples with an objection to ultrasound technology. The normal range for the speed of the baby's heartbeat is between 110 and 160 bpm. Most babies sit closer to the high end of this range early in the pregnancy. The overall rate of the baby's heart is not so important at the routine check-up as long as it is consistent and within range. It usually doesn't mean anything if, for example, one week it might be 125 bpm and the next visit 145 bpm. On one visit your baby could be sleeping, and awake the next. The most reassuring thing is knowing the heart rhythm is there and within range, and some providers will simply put a tick in this box rather than write a number during a check-up. The more detailed way to get information about your baby's heart rhythm is to use a continuous monitor or CTG (cardiotocograph) for 15 minutes or more to see the changes in the pattern over time (see page 79). This is often used in labour, but also may be used antenatally if there are concerns after a routine check-up.

Position

This is the way the baby is lying in your uterus. Head down is referred to as cephalic (Ceph for short). Bottom down is called breech (Br). Sideways is called transverse (Trans). Sometimes we write which side the baby's back is on, with either an 'R' or 'L' to signify right or left. The side with the back on it is usually where it is easier to hear the heartbeat. If we are feeling particularly confident with our assessment, or cheating with an ultrasound, we might also write if the baby is trending anterior or posterior, with the position of the spine and back of the baby's head. Occipitoanterior or 'OA' is the better way for the baby to be positioned for birth. Occipitoposterior or 'OP' is more difficult. Most of the time before labour though, the back of the baby's head is towards the side, called occipitotransverse or 'OT'. These positions often change from visit to visit, and during labour, so don't be too alarmed if your baby is posterior at a few visits.

Engagement

This refers to how deeply the baby's head is sitting down into your pelvis. The doctor or midwife will feel on either side above the pubic bone and press down to feel the baby's head. Traditionally, engagement of the head is measured as 'fifths' above or below the pubic bone. If we can feel under the baby's head, it is not engaged, or 5/5 above. If we can feel most of the head, but not under it, this is 4/5 above. If only the widest part of the head can be felt, this is 3/5 above. If only the back of the head is felt (but easily felt) this is 2/5 above, which is about as low as the head will get before labour in most women. Generally, the head will get lower and lower from around 36 weeks on. It is not unusual for the head not to engage before labour, especially in women who have had a few babies already.

Urine

Women are usually advised to send at least one urine sample off to the lab at the start of pregnancy to exclude any chronic urinary infections or other concerns. During the pregnancy, you'll generally be asked to provide a urine sample if something is not quite right, for example if you feel like an infection is starting, or have vague symptoms to suggest this, such as pains out towards your hips or strong tightenings. We also like to check your urine if your blood pressure is elevated, as the urine may show the higher protein levels associated with preeclampsia (see page 135).

Weight

While some women like to get on the scales every visit, routine weight checks have become an old-fashioned thing in most pregnancies for women in a normal weight range. Weight is important as a baseline at the start of the pregnancy. Normal weight gain is very variable and can be anywhere between 8 kg and 20 kg for women starting at a healthy weight. You should really only be asked to step on the scales routinely if your weight is at the higher or lower end of the healthy range. Some places, such as midwife-run birth centres or remote hospitals, may also have policies about safe upper weight limits for delivery. This can be due to complications if an operating theatre or anaesthetic were to be required. Obesity in pregnancy is a growing issue in Australia, and there are all sorts of things being done by health services and the government to support healthy eating, exercise and motivational support.

What I'm really thinking . . .

Putting on weight

I felt self-conscious as my clothes started to feel tight and uncomfortable. I questioned if I was gaining too much weight. But then I adjusted my mindset, and focused on nourishing my body and my baby. During my second pregnancy, I felt more confident and comfortable. I had a new-found respect for my body and I wasn't as bothered by the imperfections. I created an eating plan, ensuring my diet was varied, and steered clear of foods that were processed, high in sugar or high in trans fats. I found that with eating healthily and exercising regularly, I felt better both physically and mentally. Preparing healthy meals and snacks to keep in the fridge saved me from 'emotional eating', particularly when I wanted to reach for something sugary when I was fatigued or sore.

Note: Steady weight gain during pregnancy is normal and essential for the growth and development of your baby. It is important that you do not diet while pregnant unless recommended by a healthcare professional who can provide advice and supervision, as this may have severe consequences for your unborn baby.

UNDERSTANDING THE LINGO

Doctors and midwives can start going off on tangents when talking to women about their pregnancy. In our profession, we throw around words like 'amnion', 'dilatation' and 'meconium' like they are part of everyday conversation. Below are a few terms which can help you to understand the lingo before facing the doctor or midwife.

- **Antenatal:** Refers to the time from conceiving a pregnancy up until labour. Basically, for the duration of pregnancy.
- **Postnatal:** The time after the baby is born, up until around 6 weeks.
- **Gravidity:** The total number of pregnancies a woman has had, including miscarriages, ectopics and other first trimester mishaps. This is abbreviated as the letter G.
- **Parity:** Refers to the number of pregnancies a woman has carried beyond the second trimester and given birth to. This includes all methods of birth, and is usually counted as 1 even if twins are delivered (though some practitioners will write +1 to denote multiple birth). This is abbreviated by the letter P.
- **Nulliparous:** A woman who has never given birth. This term can also refer to women who are not currently pregnant.
- **Primiparous:** A woman who is pregnant and is going to give birth for the first time.
- **Multiparous:** A woman who has given birth multiple times. This is an important distinction. A second and subsequent birth is usually a lot different to a first birth. The good news is that multiparous birth is (generally speaking) quicker and easier than primiparous birth.
- **Uterus:** Where the baby is being grown, otherwise known as your womb. Felt as that growing balloon coming up from your pubic bone to your rib cage throughout the pregnancy. The uterus is mostly made of muscle fibres in a spiral pattern. At the top it connects to the fallopian tubes, where eggs are collected. At the bottom it connects to the cervix, where menstrual blood is shed, and babies are pushed out.
- **Fetus:** This is your baby. Until your baby is born, this is the medical term for a baby inside the womb. Most doctors won't call

your baby a fetus, but you may see the word included in certain phrases, such as 'fetal heart rate' or in your ultrasound report referring to the 'estimated fetal weight'.

- Cervix: This is the opening of the uterus, and the connection into the upper vagina from the inside of the womb. It is a tubular shape when women are not pregnant, and on average is 3 cm long. It is made up of mostly collagen and elastic tissue. During pregnancy, it has to be strong enough to keep a baby in, but during birth it has to be flexible enough to let a baby out. Hormones produced during the pregnancy help this to happen. When giving birth, the cervix flattens out like a funnel and starts to open into a circle. This is called dilatation.
- Fundus: This is the top of your womb, or the roof of baby's home. It is relevant when you get your check-ups because most midwives and doctors use the measurement to this point to check that your baby is growing.
- Birth canal: Is basically referring to your vagina. This is the passage, or canal, that your baby is going to travel down to get into the world once your cervix has completely opened up. Relevant parts of the birth canal that you may end up talking about are the pelvic bones and the perineum. During birth, the upper part of the birth canal is basically a matter of getting the bony part of the baby's head to fit into the bony part of your pelvis. There is only a centimetre or two leeway in there between the edge of the pelvis and the baby's skull, so angles matter. And usually pushing really hard also matters to get baby through this part. The lower part of the birth canal is all the soft squishy stuff. At this point, not pushing too hard is more important. When the doctor or midwife says 'stop pushing' or 'breathe', it is because the baby is coming through this part.
- Perineum: This is the area between the opening of your vagina, and the opening of your anus. This is made up of skin, collagen and muscles which move outwards like a spider's web to surround the vagina, the anus and reach across to the bony part of your groin. The total distance of the perineum when not stretched in labour is variable, but generally only between 2–4 cm. It is designed to stretch in labour, and it is stretchier in some more than others.

There are some things that you can do to condition your perineum before birth (see page 127). Don't be too disappointed if this part splits during labour, as it is also designed to be pretty forgiving with tearing and will usually heal up just fine.

- Placenta: A very versatile and fascinating organ that shares the womb with your baby. It is the thing that connects the baby to the mother and allows all the transfer of oxygen, nutrients, waste products out, water, hormones and a million other things to happen, all without mother and baby's blood even touching. It is essentially doing most of the stuff that the baby's lungs, liver, stomach and kidneys will need to do once it is in the outside world. Yet it can be safely expelled within minutes of the birth. Placentas can also be the cause of problems either before or after birth. Reactions to the placenta from patients are as variable as 'don't show it to me, just put it in the bin' to 'please keep it fresh so I can take it home and eat it'. The medical name for the tissue in the placenta is chorion.
- The membranes: The thin lining coming off the placenta, containing all the fluid, the baby and filling up to press against the walls of the womb. It is like a water balloon, which gets bigger as the baby does. This lining is called the amniotic membranes.
- Umbilical cord: The connection between the baby and the placenta. It comes out of the baby's belly button and joins onto the top of the placenta. It is basically a bridge to allow the baby to pump all of its blood back and forth to the placenta for everything described above. Babies need their umbilical cord when they are on the inside, the very definition of a lifeline. When the baby is out, all the miracles of birth happen and the vessels close in the umbilical cord. Blood stops pulsing through it within minutes of birth, allowing it to be safely cut.
- Amniotic fluid: Is commonly referred to as 'the waters'. This is all the fluid that surrounds the baby inside the womb. Another medical name for this fluid is 'liquor' pronounced 'lye-kor'. The amniotic fluid is not a fixed volume, and will change volume throughout the pregnancy, usually reaching a peak in the early third trimester. The fluid is mostly made up of urine made from the kidneys of the baby, which is then swallowed by the baby and

absorbed back into the bloodstream. This fluid is transferred back and forth across the placenta. The amount of fluid around the baby can be an indication of your health, the baby's health and how healthy the placenta is. Abnormalities of fluid volume, and what happens when you lose the fluid, is discussed on pages 141–2.

- **Amniotomy:** Also called 'artificial rupture of the membranes' or abbreviated as 'ARM'. This is where somebody breaks the waters for you rather than letting it happen naturally during labour. This is often done to speed up a slow labour, or deliberately induce a woman into labour.
- **Meconium:** Is sometimes seen in the fluid after the waters break. It usually has a brown to dark green colour. Meconium is basically the baby's first bowel movement, but inside the womb. It isn't smelly and is sterile (has no bacteria in it), and is made up of digested cells from the lining of the baby's intestines. Meconium is common, and can be a natural sign of baby's maturity, especially if it is overdue. It can also be a sign of stress on the baby, so the doctor and midwife will comment on it if seen, and usually suggest some extra precautions in labour. In a hospital environment, it will also be a reason that a paediatrician may be recommended to be present at the birth, just in case. If meconium is seen, it could be that the baby freaked out and pooped itself. When the baby is born, we try to avoid it breathing meconium into its lungs and will often recommend immediately suctioning the airway to avoid 'meconium aspiration syndrome', a term which sounds more professional than 'baby poop in the lungs'.
- **Vernix:** Is a creamy white paste that will often be seen covering the baby's skin at birth, and particularly common if the baby comes a few weeks early. It is made up of shed cells of the skin which form a fatty coating on the surface. It is a normal, healthy thing thought to be important for helping baby slide through the birth canal, and also provides a bit of a barrier from bacteria and potentially heat loss. In most cases, there is no rush to wash it off baby after birth. Think of it like baby moisturiser. In old medical textbooks, it is called 'vernix caseosa', which is Latin for 'cheesy varnish', a pretty funny, but also kind of accurate, description.

- **Labour:** Is a word that means hard work. During birth, this refers to the time when your body will be doing a lot of hard work. It can be defined differently by patients and doctors or midwives. On average, it lasts about 12 hours for first babies and gets quicker the more you do it, but is very variable. That friend of yours who was in labour for days and days was probably feeling it. If you try to tell them they weren't in labour, you will hear just how wrong you are. In strict medical terms, though, labour is defined as contractions associated with a change in the cervix over time. This is sometimes more diplomatically referred to as 'active labour'. Labour pains which aren't causing the cervix to change can be referred to as 'spurious labour' or 'the latent phase'.
- **Contractions:** This is when the uterus squeezes to push the baby out. Remember that the uterus is basically a giant muscle and, like any muscle, it is designed to create force. This force is used to help your baby to be pushed down onto your cervix during labour. Like a muscle, if it squeezes really hard it can get sore. The main difference with this muscle is that you have no real control over how strong and how frequent these contractions are. In general, when you are in labour, contractions come every 3 minutes or so, and last for up to 60 seconds. Sometimes, your doctor or midwife will use medication to increase or slow down the rate of contractions during birth. Contractions that are short, mild and usually painless are often called 'tightenings' (or Braxton Hicks) and are more common when you are not in labour.
- **Dilatation:** This is another medical word for your cervix stretching open as the baby comes through. The distance that you are 'dilated' is usually described in centimetres and assessed by feel when the doctor or midwife checks inside with their fingers. The average distance across a full-grown baby's head in a good position is about 9–10 cm. This is why people always refer to 'full dilatation' as 10 cm, but in reality, it is as open as your cervix needs to be to let the baby out. Because this distance is assessed by feel, it is very subjective – one person's 4 cm is very easily another person's 6 cm. When a woman is working really hard in labour, every centimetre counts. There is nothing more demoralising than being told by a new midwife or doctor coming onto shift that their cervix hasn't changed (or sometimes has shrunk back).

Ideally, it should be the same person doing checks for dilatation to avoid this discrepancy.

- **Oxytocin:** This is the hormone that makes your uterus contract during labour. It is made by a gland in the middle of your brain called the pituitary. It naturally comes in surges during labour, but is also stimulated by breastfeeding, and from sexual intimacy and orgasm. This is why it is often referred to as the 'love drug'. Conversely, when administered artificially via a drip to speed up or induce labour, it can get a bit of a bad rap, even though oxytocin given this way is actually chemically identical to the hormone produced by your brain. The way it is administered, the amount given and the timing of it are not the same as nature and the reason it has the potential to cause trouble. It is also a godsend for some women, whose uterus needs a good jolt of energy to get back on track.
- **CTG:** This stands for cardiotocograph, a machine with two circular sensors that are strapped to the woman's tummy with big elastic bands. One sensor picks up the baby's heartbeat, using a type of ultrasound technology. The other sensor detects contractions of the uterus. The machine then prints out lines that tell us about changes in the heart pattern of the baby over time. This is often referred to as a trace. CTGs are commonly used in labour but are also used to reassure us about babies who may be at risk of stress at any point during the third trimester.

ADDITIONAL ROUTINE TESTS

THE MORPHOLOGY ULTRASOUND

Traditionally known as 'when you get to find out the gender', the morphology ultrasound is recommended at around 20 weeks of the pregnancy (about halfway). If you are only going to have one ultrasound during your pregnancy, this is probably the most useful time to get it. It is a long ultrasound, usually taking around 30 minutes. Besides confirming the baby's gender (if you want them to), the sonographer will also systematically check all of the baby's major organs and structures.

Occasionally, a morphology ultrasound will pick up a major abnormality in the baby's development, which would require a difficult discussion with an obstetrician or paediatrician about the implications of continuing the pregnancy.

Most of the time, however, nothing unusual is found. Even if they do find something, it is important to have a discussion with your care provider before you worry too much. There are a lot of things that may be reported on morphology ultrasound that can end up having no health implications for your baby or the birth (and may even disappear by the end of the pregnancy) but are still important to be aware of.

I have listed a few things below that may show up on a report which are reasonably common to see and may end up being nothing much to worry about. As every case is different, a discussion with an obstetrician will clarify any extra monitoring or tests that may need to be done.

- Choroid plexus cyst: The choroid plexus creates the protective fluid inside the brain and around the spinal cord (called cerebrospinal fluid). Cysts are thought to occur naturally during brain development, and in most cases will have disappeared by 32 weeks. They are reported, if found, because they have a very small association with chromosomal abnormalities, which we now have much better tests to exclude. (A related but thankfully far less common finding is hydrocephalus, which is when too much fluid forms around the brain.)

- Dilated renal pelvis: The renal pelvis is where the baby's kidney first collects urine before it travels down into the bladder. When this is dilated, it does not necessarily mean there is anything wrong with the kidney or bladder, but most obstetricians will recommend checking this again in the third trimester. This is because in some cases it could be a sign of vesico-ureteric reflux, which is where some urine flows backwards towards the kidney during urination and can put infants at higher risk of kidney infections or other problems in early life. Less commonly, it can be a sign of a blockage between the kidney and bladder, which may need to be checked more urgently after birth.
- Echogenic focus: An echogenic focus is a bright spot on the ultrasound due to a higher than average density of tissue. This can be detected in a number of different organs. Many of these are transient variations in development and will often not be found if the ultrasound is repeated in the third trimester. In some cases, an echogenic focus can be a sign of a chromosomal problem (called a soft marker, because the association is low) but, as discussed above, we now have better tests to provide reassurance about chromosomal issues. Occasionally, an echogenic focus may give a warning about something which could need attention after birth, like a section of the bowel being too tight. Rarely, an echogenic focus represents an abnormal growth.
- Single umbilical artery: The umbilical cord usually has two arteries and one vein. The arteries carry blood to the placenta, and the vein carries blood away. Usually, a single umbilical artery is a variant where the two arteries fuse before the baby's belly button and continue as one. This happens in as many as 1 in 100 pregnancies. Most of the time, the baby will still develop normally and be healthy at birth. When there is a single umbilical artery, the possibility of another organ system developing unusually is higher. If the rest of the morphology scan is thought to be normal, then you can be reasonably reassured that this association is not there, but you may be offered another more detailed ultrasound to double-check the baby during the pregnancy. Single umbilical arteries do increase the chance of baby not growing enough, so additional checks later in the pregnancy will usually be suggested.

- **Low-lying placenta:** This is another very common finding, which may end up not being a problem at all. It certainly should be checked again closer to the birth to make sure that it is out of the way though.

Other things that can be identified on a morphology ultrasound are true developmental problems that may be treatable after birth. In a lot of cases, this early warning about the baby's health allows for specialist advice and preparation for a baby who may need additional care and occasionally surgical correction after birth.

On the rare occasion that I have met a couple who objected to having a morphology scan, the most common explanation for their choice (besides a fear of theoretical effects of ultrasound on the baby) is that they 'would love the baby and want to keep it – no matter what'. I can see the positive sentiment in this. To these couples, I ask: 'What if knowing about a health concern for the baby before the birth could potentially save its life?' Ultrasounds may be a little bit like spying on the mysteries of nature, but nature can be cruel sometimes.

What I'm really thinking . . .

The morphology ultrasound

For me, the morphology ultrasound was the most exciting of the scans. I will always remember when our sonographer wrote down the sex of our firstborn and gave it to us at the end of the morphology scan. My husband and I went and sat at the beach and opened it together – we just laughed hysterically as we couldn't believe that we were actually having a baby!

THE GLUCOSE TOLERANCE TEST (GTT)

Even early in the pregnancy, most patients are aware of 'that sugar drink' test. It must be one of those things that everyone who has ever had a pregnant friend has heard about. Of all the tests done routinely in a pregnancy, this is probably the one people are least excited to do. The official name for it is a glucose tolerance test. Basically, you go to the blood collector without having breakfast (fasted), then you have to scull a drink containing 75 g of glucose (the equivalent of one and a half chocolate bars). You need to stay in the waiting room for over 2 hours and you get not one, not two, but three needles for your trouble.

Glucose tolerance testing is an important screening test in pregnancy and diagnoses a condition known as gestational diabetes mellitus (GDM). To some degree, it is a normal thing for your blood sugar levels to be a bit higher when you are pregnant. Your body is focusing on making another person, and doing that takes energy. Having a good supply of sugar available for the baby is a positive thing in this regard.

In some women, the signals go a little bit overboard, and too much sugar is made available in the bloodstream. This is partly a response which is out of their control, due to hormones being pumped out by the placenta. There are some personal factors that make it a bit more likely though. Risk factors for developing gestational diabetes during pregnancy include:

- Higher maternal age: women over 30 years are at higher risk.
- A family history of type 2 diabetes or gestational diabetes.
- Being overweight.
- Cultural backgrounds including Aboriginal and Torres Strait Islander, Indian, Chinese and Middle Eastern.

As a general medical term, diabetes refers to having higher than normal blood sugar. In pregnancy, we add the word gestational to indicate that it is due to the pregnancy. Around 8 per cent of women are diagnosed with gestational diabetes. Most of the time, blood sugar levels return to normal after the pregnancy. If you get diabetes in pregnancy, you have a 50 per cent chance of getting it later in life, particularly if you don't look out for the other lifestyle factors that contribute to diabetes.

Usually, the glucose tolerance test (GTT) is done between weeks 26 and 28. Most of the time, gestational diabetes doesn't develop until the third trimester, when the placenta and baby start rapidly increasing in size. Depending on any risk factors you have, or if you have had diabetes in pregnancy before, your doctor may suggest doing the test early in the pregnancy as well, to make sure you don't get the condition early. These lucky women get to do the test twice in their pregnancy.

Of course, there are some women who have diabetes before they get pregnant. These women clearly don't have to take the test, but they also have quite a few additional challenges. If you have diabetes outside of pregnancy, it is very important that you have a talk with your doctor about planning the pregnancy before you conceive.

Tips for when you have the glucose tolerance test

- You can sip on water during the test.
- You'll be waiting at the pathology clinic for at least 2 hours, so take a book to keep you entertained while you wait.
- Take a snack to have once the testing has finished as you'll most likely be hungry.

What happens if my GTT comes back high?

Firstly, try not to be too concerned because this is only a screening test. Diabetes is not an all-or-nothing thing. Where you draw the line for 'normal' is a bit of a grey zone. If you make it too low, a lot of people will be unnecessarily worried without any serious risk. If you make it too high, some people will miss out on treatment that could improve the outcome of the disease.

There is good evidence that treating even mild gestational diabetes can improve the outcome of a birth for both baby and mother. For this reason, in Australia, we tend to diagnose it at a fairly low threshold. Using current guidelines, up to 1 in 10 women will be given the diagnosis of gestational diabetes. Some would argue that 1 out of 10 is too many, but not everybody with GDM is going to have to take medication and, if monitored and controlled, it is unlikely to have a major impact on your birth experience.

If your result comes back in a high range, you will likely be asked to see a diabetic educator. Some hospitals have special antenatal clinics dedicated to women with GDM. The goal is to provide information about diabetes and get you monitoring your blood sugar levels. This requires the use of a glucometer, a machine that can read blood sugar from a pin-prick drop of blood. You will be asked to do this four times a day (on waking, and after every main meal) and record the numbers in a diary so that the doctor or diabetic educator can help you see what the trend in your sugar is over days and weeks. For a lot of women with GDM, this is as much as they will need to do because, with good advice and a few changes in what you eat and how often, it is very possible to keep sugars in the normal range without medication. This is called diet-controlled GDM, though other lifestyle changes, such as increasing exercise, will also help to manage levels.

If your blood sugar levels are consistently outside the normal range, it may be suggested that you start medication. This can either be an oral tablet, called metformin, or a direct injection of insulin either once at night, or with every meal. Modern insulin delivery devices are very simple to use. While an unintentional overdose is extremely unlikely, some women still worry that these drugs could be harmful for their baby. Realistically, there is more risk of harm to the baby from having high sugar levels than there is from the medication used to lower blood sugar.

There are a couple of other changes to your pregnancy management that will be suggested if you have gestational diabetes. You may be advised to have an extra ultrasound midway through the third trimester, often at around 32–34 weeks, to check that baby is not too big or too small, and that your placenta is still working properly. It may also be suggested that you consider an induced labour, either at the time you are due, or even in the week before your due date, depending on how well managed your sugar levels are.

How can gestational diabetes affect my baby or the birth?

The most common possibility is that the baby grows bigger than average (called macrosomia). I discuss big babies on page 145, but it is particularly important with diabetic mothers, because the baby can grow in a disproportionate way. This means the body and shoulders can be larger relative to the head, which may be normal size. This leads to a labour risk called shoulder dystocia (page 208), where the head is out, but the doctor or midwife cannot easily get the baby's body to follow.

Conversely, with severe diabetes, the baby can be too small. This is potentially even more concerning, because it can indicate that the placenta is not functioning well. If this is the case, usually there are other signs as well, such as abnormal blood flow in the umbilical cord, or low levels of fluid around the baby. Think of the placenta as a temporary organ that has a lifespan of around 9 months. This organ lifespan can be shortened due to severe diabetes, which can lead to placental failure. This is more common in women who have diabetes before pregnancy, but is also a risk for gestationally diabetic women. Diabetes can also cause the fluid levels around the baby to become too high (called polyhydramnios).

For these reasons, women with diabetes are usually offered an induced labour. Even with an average-sized baby, there is a small increase in the risk of stillbirth for women with diabetes who go past their due date. This risk is very small, but enough to warrant offering induction. The decision to be induced can be a difficult one for many women, and often the most disappointing part about being diagnosed with gestational diabetes. For women who don't want to be induced, especially if sugar control is good and the baby is normal size, it is not unreasonable to wait for natural labour, but cautiously. Your doctor will generally offer you some increased monitoring of the baby, to make sure that the baby stays in good condition. This may mean having regular heartbeat monitoring for the baby, or another ultrasound if you are overdue.

During labour, you may be advised to have increased monitoring of the baby's heart, as well as your blood sugar. Some hospitals may suggest using a continuous heart monitor for the baby. If your sugars get too high, you may even need to be on an insulin infusion through an IV line.

Babies born to mothers with diabetes can occasionally have trouble keeping their own blood sugar stable at birth. Because of this, the baby will need a little bit of extra attention, and there is a greater chance the baby may have to be monitored in the nursery. Paediatricians refer to these babies as the 'infant of a diabetic mother', and are aware of a range of other temporary challenges that the baby may face.

There is a balance here between the treatment of the condition to avoid bad outcomes, and not interfering too much so that it ruins the experience of the birth. It is important to have a discussion about the GTT with your doctor and midwife before doing it. There can be a lot of fear about what a positive result might mean but, usually, it is not a big deal and you will get extra support throughout the pregnancy if the results are high.

What I'm really thinking:

Being diagnosed with GDM

I never imagined I would be diagnosed with gestational diabetes. I felt utterly exhausted in those early weeks of pregnancy and experienced frequent nausea, but nothing, I thought, that was out of the ordinary. (That said, looking back, I did have some occasional tingling in my hands and feet.) I was in complete shock when I got my results. I didn't understand how I could have gestational diabetes when I am quite a healthy and active person.

I was given a huge amount of information about what to eat, and I had to monitor my blood sugar levels on waking and after meals, all of which felt overwhelming at first. I also had more frequent check-ups. Although it took time to get used to, I found that with support and guidance from my doctor and midwives, I could confidently make alterations to my lifestyle to reduce the risk factors associated with gestational diabetes.

One of my main concerns was that I wouldn't be able to give birth the way I hoped to, but in the end I had a vaginal birth, just as I had planned. I was monitored while in hospital (as was my baby) and during my postpartum period, but my blood sugar levels have since returned to normal.

Emily, mum of one

David 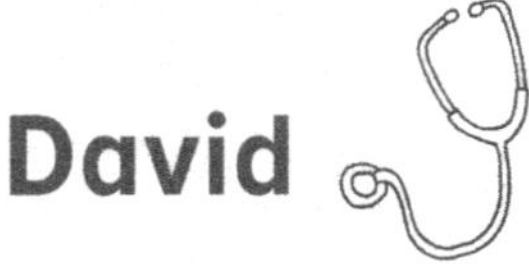

FULL BLOOD, IRON STORES AND ANAEMIA

Anaemia means that your body is running low on the stuff your blood needs to carry oxygen. This is called haemoglobin (Hb) and is inside the red blood cells. The most important nutrients required to make new blood cells are iron, folate and vitamin B12.

During pregnancy, your body actually creates more blood than normal. However, the blood is more diluted because you are also carrying a lot of extra fluid when you are pregnant (ask your ankles and wrists about that . . .) and a lot of the blood is redirected to the placenta for baby. By the end of your pregnancy, a third of your blood volume passes through your uterus and placenta each minute.

Even though all pregnant women make more blood than usual, it is also very common for your blood count to start to trend towards the anaemic range. Your body will use a lot more iron than it did prior to getting pregnant. It is almost more common than not to see a level of iron deficiency by the third trimester, especially in women who have not routinely been taking a supplement.

The symptoms of anaemia are pretty much the symptoms of pregnancy, which makes detecting anaemia without a routine blood test more challenging. You may feel any of the following:

- Easily fatigued or generally less energetic.
- Breathless without doing much to exert yourself (even just while sitting).
- Light-headed on standing or with a sudden change in temperature.

In over 90 per cent of cases, if you are becoming anaemic during pregnancy, your doctor will advise increasing iron replacement. This is usually started with a dedicated iron tablet (more than what is in the typical pregnancy multivitamin). The iron tablet can then be increased to twice a day if needed. The most common side effects are constipation or an upset stomach. There is no point in taking more than two iron supplements a day, as there is only so much your body will let you absorb in 24 hours. If iron deficiency is not able to be corrected with tablets, your doctor may recommend an iron infusion through the vein, or iron injections into the muscle. These are convenient ways to quickly boost your iron stores, but they do come with some minor risks of an adverse reaction.

Sometimes, anaemia will be due to other nutritional factors that can be corrected, or genetic issues such as thalassaemia, which may need further testing to see if there will be any impact on the baby. With typical iron-deficiency anaemia, the risks for the baby are low unless the anaemia is severe, and most of the need to correct blood counts comes from improving the symptoms of anaemia for the mother and getting them prepared for birth with as normal a blood count as possible.

BLOOD GROUP ANTIBODY SCREENING

Most people have heard of the idea of a blood type. The common blood types A, B, AB and O are only one basic group – there are many other different typing systems for blood. The other common one that people have often heard of is whether they are positive or negative. This actually refers to a specific typing of blood called Rhesus D.

When it comes to pregnancy, the baby has a 50 per cent chance of inheriting blood types (for all the different systems) from either the mother or the father. If the baby inherits a blood type that is different to the mother, there is a small chance that the mother's immune system may recognise this blood type as foreign and may then begin to attack the baby's blood.

This requires two things to happen:

1. The mother must be exposed to the baby's blood, which is reasonably common in labour and birth, but usually requires a 'sensitising event' to occur during the antenatal part of the pregnancy, such as trauma to the abdomen, or a placental bleed.
2. The type of blood group of the baby must create an antibody from the mother, which is able to cross the placenta and have an effect on the blood of the baby.

In Australia, any woman who is a negative blood group is offered injections of 'anti-D' during pregnancy to prevent this phenomenon of making antibodies against the baby's blood. Anti-D is actually a small amount of the antibody that we don't want the mothers to make, and is derived from donor blood. The principle of action is like a reverse immunisation.

There are a number of other blood types that the baby may have for which we do not yet have a system of preventing mothers making antibodies. The blood group antibody screening tests offered to pregnant women during pregnancy help to screen for these less common types, as well as the 1 in 7 who are negative blood groups.

If you are found to have a minor blood group antibody as a result of this screening, you may need to have additional blood tests during the pregnancy to ensure that concentrations of the antibody are not increasing. You may also need to have additional ultrasound screening in the third trimester to make sure that the baby is not becoming affected by these antibodies. It is important, however, to note that some minor blood group antibodies are completely harmless.

Can I go to the dentist while pregnant?

Yes, a visit to the dentist while pregnant is safe. Let your dentist know that you are pregnant, and they will avoid undertaking any unnecessary testing, such as X-rays. Having a regular check-up and clean is safe and beneficial as dental hygiene is important, particularly during pregnancy.

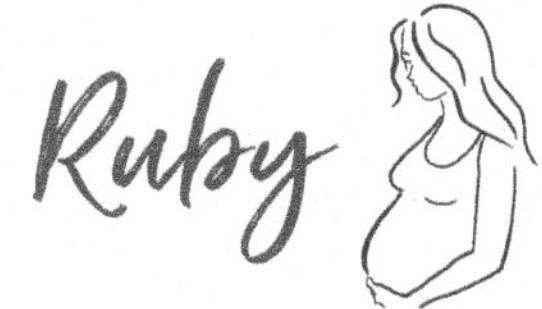

FEELING WELL IN THE SECOND TRIMESTER

If you are wondering why you don't have that pregnancy glow they all talk about, you are certainly not alone. For some of us, this glow never comes, the fatigue lingers the whole way through, and the back pain and leg cramps keep you wondering when the so-called 'honeymoon period' is officially going to begin!

SLEEP

Those who have children will continue to offer the advice to 'sleep now, before baby comes'. However, as you get further along in the pregnancy sleeping may be uncomfortable. Sleeping on your side may be difficult, particularly if you are usually a belly sleeper. There can be several other reasons why you may not be getting a good night's sleep:

- Pelvic pain.
- Heartburn (see page 105).
- Nasal congestion.
- Vivid dreams or nightmares.
- Frequent trips to the bathroom.

Then there's the issue of dealing with a belly the size of a netball! In the summer, heat may also play a role in a disturbed and unpleasant night's sleep.

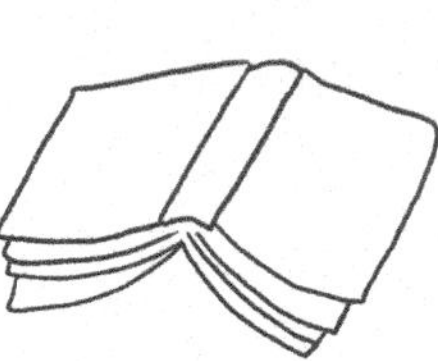

Tips for better sleep:

- Use a pillow between your legs for support when lying on your side.
- Use a rolled-up towel or folded pillow propped next to your belly to avoid rolling. This is particularly helpful when you reach the third trimester as your stomach grows larger and the weight naturally makes you fall forward, which can result in pelvic pain. Propping a towel or pillow on your side, between your legs and behind you to support your back can be an inexpensive option to get more comfortable.
- Avoid foods that aggravate heartburn, such as spicy foods, caffeinated drinks and some acidic foods, including tomatoes and citrus fruits. Propping yourself up on pillows can ease heartburn and indigestion.
- Choose comfortable, loose-fitting sleepwear.
- If you are fortunate enough and time permits, a siesta during the day can help with fatigue and allow you to catch up on a few extra hours of rest.

What I'm really thinking . . .

Getting a good night's sleep

Being a belly sleeper, all I wanted to do was lie on my stomach. I realised that wasn't going to happen, considering my belly was the size of a watermelon, and I would have settled with getting comfortable on my back. But when I did try, it lasted just a few seconds before breathlessness and heartburn came rushing onto the scene. Propping pillows up behind me so I was slightly upright helped relieve some of these symptoms. In the end I discovered I was most comfortable lying on my side with a pillow propped around me. (And the greatest feeling ever was lying on the beach and digging a hole in the sand to place my large belly in – bliss!)

David

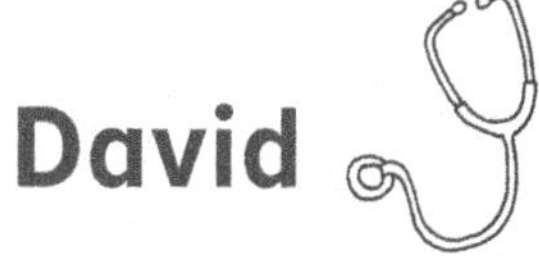

NATURAL THERAPIES

Very broadly, most alternative therapies suggested by qualified practitioners are not known to be harmful for pregnant women or their babies. The typical concern of many doctors is that they are not known to be safe either. Prescription medications are subject to strict regulations and review regarding safety in pregnancy. Most natural remedies are not subject to the same rules, though many have been studied extensively. It is worth considering other exposures during the extraction of the active ingredients, such as heavy metals or alcohol. It is also important to know there are some natural remedies which are definitely known to have important interactions on other prescription drugs. They may also have an impact on liver metabolism or the ability for the blood to clot. If you are ingesting a natural remedy, it is wise to find out precisely what is in it. This knowledge may be useful for your doctor. For example, fish oil is known to thin the blood, and St John's Wort alters liver metabolism. Some herbs, such as pennyroyal, dong quai or black cohosh, are associated with uterine contractions and miscarriage. Some well established natural remedies will likely be happily supported by your care provider in the right circumstances, such as ginger for first trimester nausea, or raspberry leaf tea from the third trimester. With green tea, keep in mind the possible caffeine content.

With physical manipulations, so long as the practitioner is not doing these directly on the baby, it is unlikely to be a concern. For example, if any practitioner offered to physically turn a breech baby with direct pressure outside the hospital environment, I would be concerned. Also, keep in mind that your collagen and joints are particularly soft during pregnancy. Spinal and joint manipulations may need a gentler touch to avoid harm. Massage, osteopathy and acupuncture treatments may also be offered in a seated, leaning forward position, or lying on your side during the third trimester to avoid direct pressure on the baby. Acupuncture is safe to have while pregnant, although there is no scientific evidence to suggest it is beneficial. However, anything that promotes relaxation and a feeling of wellbeing can only be a good thing.

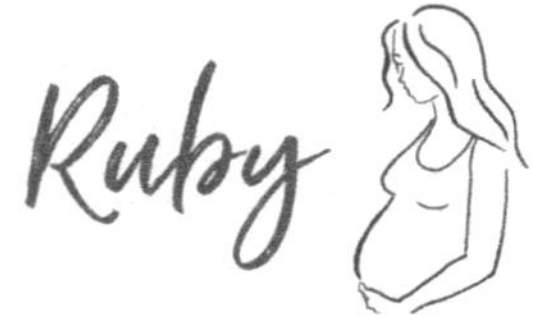

EXERCISE DURING PREGNANCY

It isn't uncommon for pregnant women to question whether they can safely continue with their regular exercise routine. If you do not normally exercise but have decided that now is the time to start, make sure it is a gentle regime.

Can I continue to exercise for the whole 9 months?

Yes. Exercise is extremely beneficial for our physical and mental wellbeing, and it may help to relieve constipation, fatigue and cramping, and prevent excessive weight gain. Exercising is also a good way to keep your heart healthy and improve muscle tone, which can ease any pain or discomfort you are feeling, particularly as you come into the second and third trimester.

What type of exercise is ideal?

The best and safest forms of exercise during pregnancy, particularly if you didn't have an exercise regime prior to becoming pregnant, are walking, water aerobics or low-impact aerobics, swimming and light weight training.

What should I do differently?

- Implement pelvic floor exercises into your regular regime.
- Avoid dehydration. Make sure you drink plenty of water during and after exercising.
- Warm-up exercises, stretching and cooling down can be beneficial in helping blood flow and avoiding injury.
- Be cautious when exercising in hot or humid climates. It is best to exercise in the morning or afternoon.
- As you enter the second trimester, you may feel more comfortable avoiding exercises that involve lying flat on your back. You may feel faint due to the pressure of the uterus on a major vein in the abdomen that can interfere with blood flow back to the heart. Propping yourself up may be ideal as your belly begins to grow.

It is important to avoid activities that may cause injury or have a higher risk of falling. Keep a distance from the extreme sports such as horse-riding, skiing, contact sports or other activities that are high risk. Deep-sea diving should be avoided during pregnancy.

What I'm really thinking . . .

Staying active

For me, exercise wasn't just about clarity of mind and keeping fit, it was also about gaining confidence in my new-found body that, honestly, took a while to get used to. Finding a healthy balance between what I enjoyed doing and what my body and mood permitted proved challenging at times. Lower back pain, accompanied by pelvic pain and lingering fatigue, sometimes made exercising seem unbearable. For me, pregnancy yoga helped relieve the tension in my limbs and also quietened my mind as I struggled with heightened anxiety towards the end of my pregnancy. Yoga was also beneficial in easing back pain and allowing me to properly relax.

I would also swim a few laps a couple of times a week at the local pool. Swimming made me feel stronger and toned, and it also aided in relieving back pain and sciatica. The lightness I felt when floating was bliss, particularly in the third trimester when I was heavy and uncomfortable, and all I wanted to do was get off my swollen feet for a few moments.

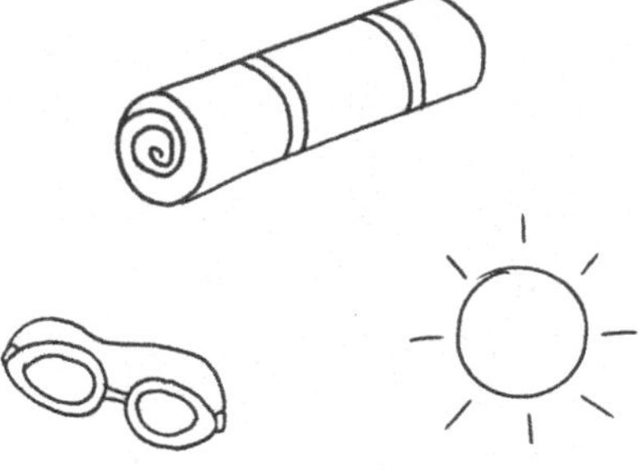

THE PELVIC FLOOR

The pelvic floor is the name for the group of muscles, tendons and ligaments that support a woman's uterus (womb), bowel and bladder. The muscles and connective tissues work together to help prevent incontinence and reduce the risk of prolapse, and also aid with sexual function. During your pregnancy, your pelvic floor is under extra pressure, so strengthening those muscles becomes very important.

To locate your pelvic floor, squeeze and lift your pelvic region inwards and upwards as if you are trying to stop wind or urine and draw your lower stomach muscles inwards. Hold for a few seconds and then feel your pelvic floor relax after the hold. As you become more confident in practising your pelvic floor exercises, increase the hold and lift for a few more seconds, and increase how many times in a row you repeat them. You can do these exercises while sitting, standing or lying down. Keep your stomach, thighs and bottom relaxed. There is no need to alter your breathing when undertaking pelvic floor exercises (don't hold your breath!). If you are unsure how to do them or have any concerns, speak with a physiotherapist.

Doing your pelvic floor exercises regularly throughout pregnancy and postpartum will help to prevent pelvic floor issues such as incontinence and prolapse. It is also beneficial to continue exercising your pelvic floor muscles after your baby is born, particularly when lifting your baby, coughing or sneezing. Set aside time every day.

Finding time for your pelvic floor exercises!

It isn't until you give birth that you realise the importance of your pelvic floor and how imperative it is to strengthen it during pregnancy and postpartum. I made it my mission to get into a habit of doing them daily, and I am so glad I did! The great thing about these exercises is that you can do them anywhere, at any time. If you exercise daily, simply incorporate pelvic floor exercises into your routine. If you have a long commute to work, do your 'lift and hold' at the traffic lights or on the train or bus. You can even do them while hanging out the washing, or sitting at your desk at work.

David

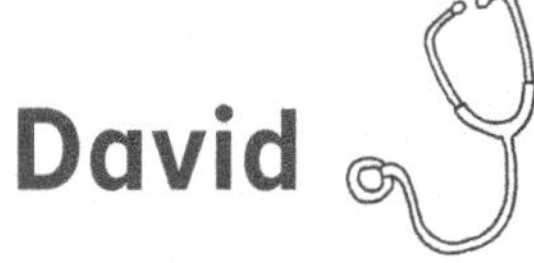

MENTAL HEALTH CONDITIONS

The second trimester is the time when many women in Australian hospitals are first formally screened for mental health concerns. An Edinburgh Depression Scale, or similar mental health questionnaire, has become a standard part of the booking-in process at most hospitals. Most GPs, obstetricians and midwives are also very alert to the importance of mental health and will have performed some level of assessment during initial discussions.

There are lots of broad labels we put on mental health conditions and behavioural states. Depression, anxiety, bipolar, psychosis, schizophrenia, ADD, OCD, PTSD . . . Women can and do fall pregnant with these as pre-existing conditions. Some women develop mental health disorders for the first time during pregnancy. Of this second group, depression and anxiety are the most common newly developing conditions during a pregnancy. Research shows that 1 in 10 women experience antenatal depression in Australia.

In the first trimester, mental health is often affected by the psychosocial changes happening in the woman's life as she adapts to the idea of going through a pregnancy. Issues with family members or domestic partners may develop if there are conflicting ideas about being pregnant. Ultimately, it is the woman who carries the baby, so she will be the centre of any emotional turmoil. During the first trimester, other physiological changes (especially morning sickness) and hormonal changes can also impact how a woman feels psychologically.

Australia has one of the lowest rates of pregnancy-related death in the world. Alarmingly, though, mental health-related conditions are one of the leading causes of death amongst Australian women during pregnancy and in the first year after the birth. Suicide, self-harm, substance abuse and domestic violence are all serious issues linked to mental health disorders. Any woman at risk should talk with her doctor, midwife, social worker, psychologist or other healthcare provider to access government-funded mental health services. Many of these are specifically designed for care during and immediately after pregnancy.

If you are experiencing feelings of anxiety, depression or low moods that won't budge, or you are feeling a lack of enjoyment in life, it is important to know that you are not alone. It's normal to start thinking (sometimes over-thinking) about your living or work arrangements. It is common to feel anxious or nervous about how life will change when this tiny human comes along. Many women say that they didn't want to appear 'ungrateful' for being pregnant or felt pressure to enjoy pregnancy although they felt otherwise. Some signs to look out for include:

- Low moods that last more than 2 weeks
- Emotions that are negatively impacting your ability to complete everyday tasks
- A lack of enjoyment or pleasure in life
- Frequently feeling overwhelmed or anxious
- Struggling to fall or stay asleep.

Discuss with your doctor how you are feeling and if you are not coping as they may suggest a treatment plan or strategies. Similar techniques in treating any form of depression and anxiety may be used to treat perinatal depression, including speaking with a trained professional such as a social worker or psychologist, using tools to help practise mindfulness to reduce anxiety, and/or medication.

Taking antidepressant medication during pregnancy

As a general rule, if you take medication due to a mental health condition and find out you are pregnant, you should not immediately stop this medication, but speak to a doctor as soon as possible. Sometimes dose adjustments or alternative medication may be suggested, but stopping medication suddenly can exacerbate mental health conditions if you are not emotionally and psychologically prepared. The most common medications taken by pregnant women for mental health are antidepressants, and particularly SSRIs or SNRIs. The risks that taking these medications will have an impact on your baby are reasonably low and manageable. Some of these relate to the chance of baby suffering withdrawal symptoms after birth, for which a plan to be prepared can help.

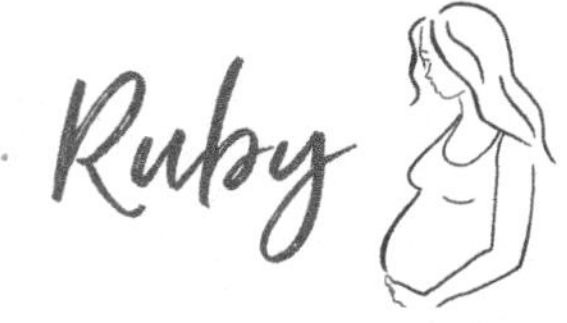

YOUR MENTAL AND EMOTIONAL HEALTH

This topic is, in my opinion, one of the most important of all, and one that is not always openly talked about. A crucial element of prenatal care is your mental wellbeing. For many women, pregnancy is an emotional time. We can go through ups and downs as we enter new phases over the 9 months, worrying about the transition from work to motherhood, our living situation, our proximity to family and friends, our relationship with our partner or even fear of giving birth.

We tend to hear about the joy of pregnancy, the anticipation women feel about becoming a mother and bringing new life into the world. Implicit in this rosy view of pregnancy is that we know what we're doing, and that we should feel positive and grateful for the entire experience, yet this couldn't be further from the truth. Pregnancy can be a minefield and we may question what we are doing, how our baby is growing and developing and if we are making the right choices along the way. I found that meeting other mothers-to-be in antenatal classes or prenatal exercise classes helped to ease my insecurities about pregnancy.

Meditation and mindfulness is a great way to reduce anxiety. I have never found it easy to meditate on my own, so I decided to try guided meditations through an app (I used Headspace). These can be incredibly helpful, and I found that practising mindfulness on a daily basis for just 5–10 minutes helped to reduce my worries, particularly in the weeks leading up to the birth.

I also had to learn to trust the advice of my doctors and midwives, which was difficult for me. But I found that once I let them in and expressed my concerns, I received a lot of ongoing support and encouragement, particularly from the midwives, who really made me feel at ease. If you are experiencing anxiety or depression during your pregnancy or the first year of motherhood, it is very important that you seek professional help. Pregnancy is such a delicate time and a huge transition for every woman.

Dealing with stress and mood swings

Waking up feeling elated and happy, then crying at the drop of a hat? You are not alone – many pregnant women know this all too well. The nausea, bloating, back pain and fatigue do not help either. You may notice that your mood swings settle during the second trimester, and then the tears may come flooding back in the lead up to your due date (I cried almost every day in the last week before I gave birth in my second pregnancy).

If you are feeling that you have high stress levels, whether they are to do with your pregnancy or not, here are a few tips that may help:

- Go for a walk in a park or out in nature – the sun exposure will boost your vitamin D levels and the fresh air will also help.
- Spend some quality time with family or friends, sharing your worries or stresses with people who you love and trust.
- Read a book or head to the movies.
- Listen to relaxation music or a favourite playlist.
- Practise mindfulness daily.
- Swim, walk, practise yoga, dance or do some other kind of low-impact exercise that you love.
- Take a warm and relaxing bath.
- Tune out from social media, which can at times portray pregnancy in an unrealistic light. Don't compare your pregnancy with others'.
- Switch off your devices. Research shows that turning off phones, laptops, TVs and other screens at night helps us to wind down and get a better night's sleep.
- Accept help and support.
- Have an honest chat with your partner. Try to help them understand how you're feeling and what your body is going through so that they can offer support.

There is a distinction between mood swings and perinatal depression and anxiety. If you are experiencing low moods that affect your daily life and functioning, or you are frequently feeling anxious, it is important to speak with your doctor or midwife. They can help you find the best support and treatment.

David

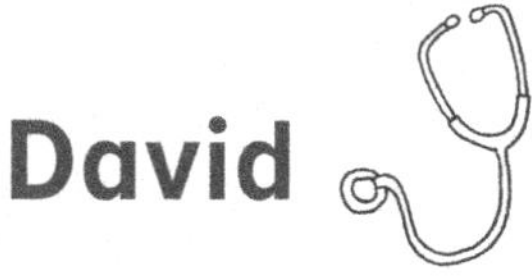

WILL STRESS HURT MY BABY?

While psychological stress is miserable for you it is not known to directly harm your baby, so if you are suffering stress or anxiety, you can cross that worry off your list.

Stress certainly has numerous effects on the body that will influence your experience of pregnancy. Sleeplessness and fatigue. Higher stress hormone levels. Poor diet or appetite (either over- or under-eating). These are all things that can be directly impacted by stress and will impact on your general wellbeing.

Inside your womb, the placenta is the physiological link between you and your baby. Emotional, spiritual and psychological links are unquantifiable with modern science, and play a part in the growing bond between you and your baby. As far as the placenta goes, there are three main things the baby needs from your body – nutrients, oxygen and the ability to get rid of waste products from metabolism. As a broad generalisation, if the placenta is functioning, the mother has to be fairly unwell for any of these three things to be compromised in a big way. There are many hormones in you that change in response to psychological stress. These include adrenaline and cortisol. There is some evidence that these hormones can have an impact on the muscle of the uterus, or the blood supply to the placenta. A lot of this is in relation to the stress of labour, and the link between a calm birthing environment and a smoother birth experience.

Prolonged stress can progress to more significant mental health concerns such as anxiety disorders or depression. The most important thing is to let people know if you are feeling significantly stressed, so they can start looking into ways to manage and reduce your stress.

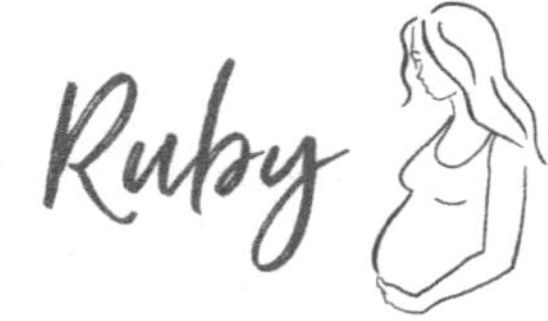

FETAL MOVEMENTS

One of the most incredible feelings is the sensation of your baby moving inside you. You may feel flutters from as early as 16 weeks, though don't be alarmed if you don't. As a first-time mother, you may not be quite sure what they feel like yet. First, it starts with flutters, then the kicks begin to feel stronger, more intense and sometimes rapid. Your baby's hiccups feel bizarre at first, then familiar as the weeks go by.

You may feel movements more often at night, when you are sitting down relaxing and more in tune with the kicking and rolling sensations. In the later stages of pregnancy, when your baby is getting much bigger and there is less room to move, you may find the movements are more rolling and wriggle sensations.

All babies are different and some tend to move more than others. Some babies move more at night or in the morning, others are active all day. If your movements are consistent with your baby's usual activity and you feel them regularly, there is no need to worry.

What I'm really thinking . . .

Feeling my baby move

There is nothing more amazing than feeling your baby dance inside you. I could never get enough of the feeling. I would worry (as all first-time mothers do) if I hadn't felt my baby move for a while, especially at night when she was typically most active. I would drink sparkling water to see if the bubbles would get her moving. I remember one time where I hadn't felt her move and was nervous that something was wrong. My husband and I got in the car and drove the back streets of Byron, the ones that were full of potholes, to see if that would get her moving. They did – and now we think back to this moment and laugh.

My baby's movements have slowed down or stopped. What should I do?

If you have noticed that your baby's movements have slowed or stopped completely, it is important to contact your midwife, doctor or the hospital as soon as possible.

Usually, the midwives will advise you to drink a cup of cold water, move around and give your tummy a little poke and prod to see if your baby moves. If there is still no movement, you will be asked to come in for monitoring. Don't worry at all if you get into the hospital and your baby starts kicking and moving around. It is always better to be sure and for you to feel at ease.

BONDING WITH YOUR BUMP

There is a tiny being growing inside of you, and some days, it may feel as though being pregnant is utterly exhausting. Try and make time to connect with your baby along the way. Everyone bonds with their baby differently during pregnancy, just as they do once baby is born, so don't be worried if you don't have an immediate connection. Here are some ways to bond with your bump:

- Massage your bump.
- Talk or sing to your baby throughout the day (your baby can hear you).
- Listen to music.
- Take photos of your growing bump throughout your pregnancy.
- Write down all the weird and wonderful things that are happening during your pregnancy i.e. cravings, kicks, feelings and emotions.
- Give your baby a nickname (we called our daughter 'Minnie').
- When baby starts kicking and moving, take a moment to enjoy the movements. This is also a lovely way for your partner to connect with your baby.
- Visualise your baby or, even better, see them on a 3D or 4D scan.

CONNECTING WITH YOUR PARTNER

If you are in an intimate relationship, when a baby comes along it is no longer just the two of you. You instantly become a team, and there are many changes that occur within those first few months. We all handle birth and recovery as best we can, then launch into a lack of sleep, while trying to master feeding (and don't forget to throw in all those raging hormones). It all takes a toll on our relationships.

During the pregnancy, it is important to spend time together as a couple and enjoy the simple things that will become somewhat of a rarity once your baby comes along.

- Do things together such as cooking dinner, going out for breakfast on the weekend, taking a trip to the beach, visiting an art gallery or spending quality time with friends and family.
- Keep the lines of communication open. Both of you are coming to terms with the fact that you are going to be parents, and talking about your joys and concerns keeps you connected.
- Make time for dates.
- Don't be afraid to have sex. It is safe for both mother and baby (see opposite).
- Take a babymoon. It could be a luxury escape or a camping trip to your favourite spot – the important thing is to spend quality time together.
- Plan and get organised together. This will ease the pressure when your baby arrives.
- Talk about things other than the pregnancy.

Is it safe to have sex during pregnancy?

While it may seem embarrassing asking your doctor or friend if you're going to hurt your unborn baby by having sex, if you are wondering about this, you are not alone. Many couples worry that sexual activity will cause harm to their unborn child; this is not the case. Sexual intercourse can continue during pregnancy unless there are complications and you have been advised otherwise. Your baby is tightly protected by your cervix and the mucus plug, and sheltered in the amniotic sac, so there is no need to be concerned.

SYMPTOMS AND SIDE EFFECTS

As the second trimester progresses, many women describe a pulling sensation 'down there': the stretching of ligaments and the enlarging of your uterus is to blame for that. It is a lot more noticeable in a first pregnancy and becomes more apparent as you near the third trimester. It may have you wondering what on earth is going on but, be assured, it is normal and all part of your baby becoming bigger and healthier as your due date draws closer.

HEARTBURN

Heartburn (acid reflux) is common in pregnancy and tends to come on during the second or third trimester. However, it may be experienced at any time during your pregnancy, and might come and go.

Heartburn is a burning-like pain caused by stomach acid moving up the oesophagus. This happens because the increase in progesterone while pregnant relaxes the stomach valve. Many women will experience heartburn for the first time while pregnant, but this will usually settle after birth.

Antacid reflux medication may be used in normal dosage. Ranitidine and esomepraze are category B, which means they have no proven harm but they should be used with caution during pregnancy.

Here are a few alternative options that you may like to consider:

- If you notice that the heartburn is worst at nighttime after a meal or when lying down, prop yourself up on a pillow while sleeping to help ease the sensation.
- Eat smaller meals more frequently.
- Avoid fatty, fried or spicy foods as these can exacerbate acid reflux symptoms.

HAYFEVER

If you are affected by allergic rhinitis, otherwise known as hayfever, you may find it worsens in pregnancy. Avoiding known allergens is the best way to reduce your symptoms. Here are some safe ways of dealing with allergic rhinitis while pregnant:

- Saline sprays and rinses.
- Steam – using a bowl and hot water with a towel over your head.
- Many non-drowsy antihistamines are category B, which means you can use them with caution during pregnancy to alleviate hayfever symptoms, especially after the second trimester.
- Over-the-counter nasal sprays are also generally safe to use while pregnant, but check with your doctor regarding specific products.

SKIN CHANGES DURING PREGNANCY

Cholasma or melasma

A blotchy or brown pigmentation on the skin during pregnancy is referred to as cholasma or melasma. You may have heard of this condition being referred to as the 'pregnancy mask'. The pigmentation affects the darker areas of the skin, on the forehead, chin and the upper lip area.

Cholasma is the overproduction of the pigment melanin from the skin cells called melanocytes. Many women develop cholasma in pregnancy due to hormonal changes, and it generally affects those with darker skin tones.

Skin pigmentation worsens with sun exposure. Wearing sunscreen and protecting your face and skin from the sun helps reduce the skin pigmentation.

You may find that the pigmentation fades substantially once the baby has arrived. In many cases, it will eventually disappear. If you are still concerned post-pregnancy, seeing a dermatologist to look at treatment options is the best approach.

Burst capillaries on the body and face are also common during pregnancy and occur due to the volume of blood moving around your body. In most cases, the capillaries subside post-pregnancy and instances where they don't can also be treated by a dermatologist.

What is the dark line down the centre of my stomach?

This dark line is called linea nigra. The melanocyte-stimulating hormone is responsible for the line developing, which may appear in the second or third trimester. You may have also noticed your nipples and other spots on your body have darkened in colour since being pregnant. This is due to the same hormones. Wondering if it will go away? The answer is yes, it does eventually fade over time. It took just under a year for the dark line on my stomach and in my belly button to finally disappear.

Pain relief medication

There may come a time in your pregnancy when you experience aches and pains such as headaches or back pain. Most of the time, there is no need for medication, just rest, hydration and time. However, if the pain is persistent, you may want the relief of pain medications.

The main class of pain medications unsuitable for pregnant women are the 'non-steroidal anti-inflammatory drugs', or NSAIDs. This includes ibuprofen, as well as some other over-the-counter drugs like diclofenac and mefamic acid. Aspirin, in pain relief doses, is also not recommended, but is used for other indications in small doses (up to 100 mg once a day compared with 300 mg two to three times a day for pain). The reason that these drugs are not recommended is that they can interfere with the levels of amniotic fluid around the baby and have a small chance of causing early closure of an important structure in the baby's cardiac circulation, the ductus venosus.

Paracetamol is generally thought to be fine in pregnancy and is usually the first line of pain relief. Opiate analgesics such as codeine, oxycodone and tramadol are not directly harmful to the baby, but can be habit-forming, which can lead to withdrawal symptoms for both mother and baby. These drugs tend to be used only for more significant pain, and if used for prolonged periods close to the birth, the baby should be watched for withdrawal. If you suffer from migraines, treating these can be a little more complicated, as some of the drugs used for migraine specifically are not recommended in pregnancy either. As with all medications, it is best to discuss with your doctor.

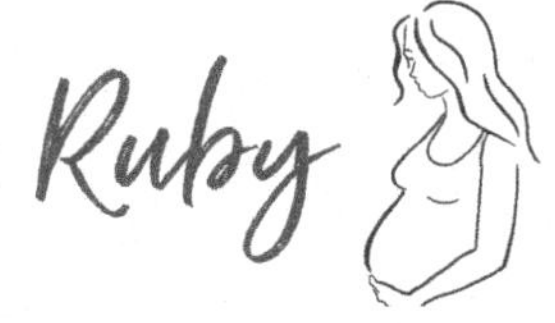

Striae or stretch marks

Stretch marks are very common and harmless. They are a result of the excess tension on the skin as your body makes room for your growing baby. Striae are commonly found on the abdomen, but you may also notice them on your thighs, bottom, breasts and upper arms. During pregnancy, they will appear as red or purplish lines, however, over time they do fade to a white or silvery grey colour.

You've probably seen the line-up of products in the chemist or beauty section that claim to 'prevent or cure' stretch marks. So far there is little (if any) evidence to suggest that they do. However, it can be a nice way to massage your tummy and bond with your baby, plus it feels very self-nurturing. If your stretch marks bother you, it is recommended that you wait until the postnatal period to seek medical advice and treatment from a dermatologist.

What I'm really thinking:

Learning to love my stretch marks

I didn't know I had stretch marks until the last few months of pregnancy. I couldn't see them clearly because my bump was in the way, but when I looked in the mirror, these purplish red lines appeared as stripes across my lower abdomen. For me, there was no escaping them (especially the second time around). No matter how often I lathered myself with oil, they still appeared. (Then there are the lucky few who, due to genetics and skin tone, manage to avoid getting them at all!) Even though developing stretch marks caused me some anxiety at times, I now consider them to be an intrinsic part of myself: they are my stripes, the stripes I earned from growing my beautiful babies.

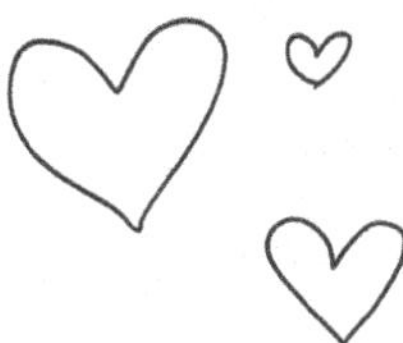

MATERNITY CLOTHES

What you need to know:

- You may not need to buy maternity clothes until the second trimester, or later.
- Ask your friends if you can borrow maternity clothes.
- Look for second-hand options such as buy/swap/sell sites on Facebook, Instagram, Gumtree and eBay.
- Choose clothes that are elastic or stretchy, such as activewear. You can pull down stretchy pants to sit under your stomach once it begins to grow larger.
- You can buy belly bands that link onto your jeans and pants, which don't cost a lot of money. These come in handy particularly in the first months of pregnancy when you can still squeeze into those jeans (at least for a little while longer) but aren't yet showing.
- If you do decide to buy maternity clothes, choose loose tops or ones with buttons so you can breastfeed down the track.

When should I buy nursing bras?

Nursing bras aren't all that glamorous, but they are incredibly comfortable. They have the support that is needed for your growing breasts, don't have any underwire and can be quite affordable.

If you have breast soreness or your breasts have already doubled in size, you might start thinking about switching from your regular bras to nursing bras before baby is born. At around 5–6 months into your pregnancy, you may decide it is time to start wearing underwire-free bras. If you do choose to buy nursing bras prior to giving birth, be aware that your breasts will increase in size once you start breastfeeding. You may decide to buy a few bras that are a size up in preparation for this. If you are not yet ready to surrender to the nursing bra, ditch the underwire and use your workout or crop bras for comfort.

David

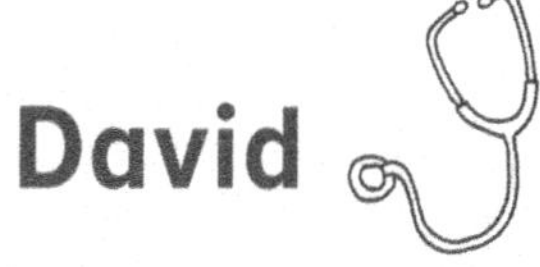

TRAVELLING WHILE PREGNANT

Travelling while pregnant up until week 32 is safe and requires no documentation. After 32 weeks, airlines ask for written consent from a doctor or midwife to give the all-clear to fly. It is a good idea to consult with your doctor or midwife if you are high-risk or are having multiples, as there may be restrictions to your travel in these cases depending on your health and circumstances. The risk of deep vein thrombosis, which is blood clotting in the leg, is greater the further along you are in your pregnancy.

Many insurance companies will not insure you if you travel after 26 weeks. If you are travelling to a developing country such as Indonesia or Thailand, it's best to visit government websites to check if there are any active health risks such as dengue fever from mosquito bites, water-borne diseases or food-borne illnesses that can pose a risk if you are pregnant.

Zika virus is dangerous for pregnant women as it may cause birth defects. It is spread via mosquitos but can also be spread via sexual intercourse with an infected person who may not even have symptoms. It is recommended that you defer travel to Zika-affected countries. If you need to travel to this area, having a discussion with your doctor is important. If your partner is travelling to an infected area, let your doctor know and practise safe sex.

What I'm really thinking . . .

Going on holiday

I was hesitant booking a holiday, particularly to a developing country where extra precautions needed to be taken. When I travelled to Bali and Fiji, I only drank bottled or filtered water, used copious amounts of natural insect repellents and ate food only from reputable restaurants. I also avoided meat and eggs to help reduce my risk of contracting food-borne illnesses.

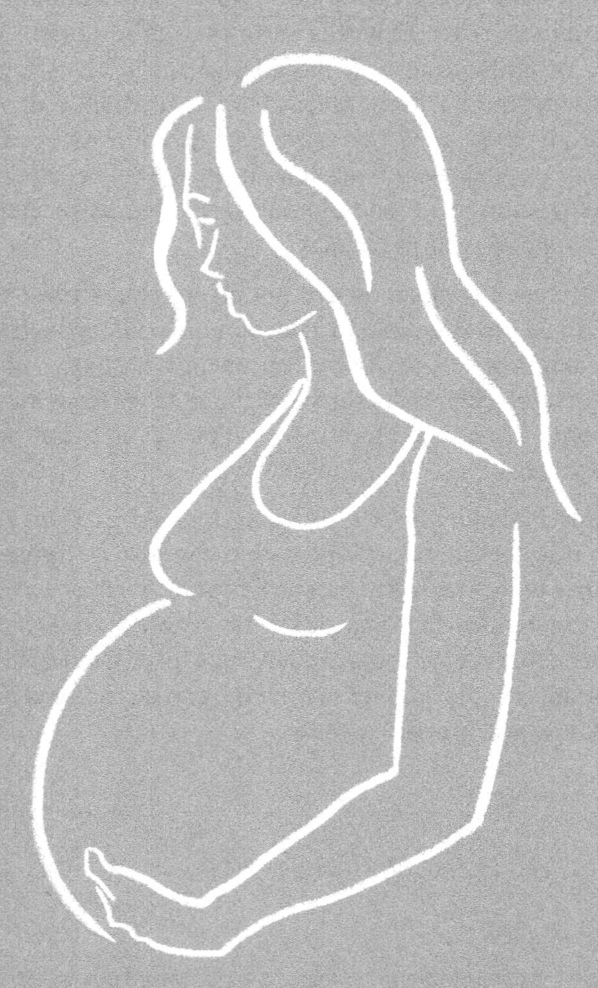

THIRD TRIMESTER

David

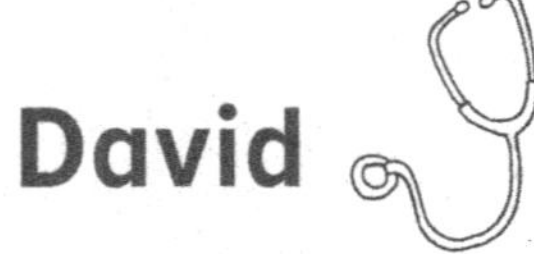

This is it: the home stretch. You got through the fatigue and nausea of the first trimester. You grew your baby large enough to survive outside the womb. Now, you have to let it get bigger and wait for it to come out. By this stage, most women are fairly confident that all checks have been done and any problems should already be on the radar. Generally, a woman in the third trimester is much more in tune with her baby. It is much more evident how the baby is lying and movements are obvious, with the baby likely establishing a movement pattern that is predictable and reassuring. A lot of women and their partners will be talking to their baby, stroking it or playing with the little limbs that may emerge as points on the bump, exploring the surface like a periscope.

What I'm really thinking . . .

The final weeks

The last weeks of pregnancy can be physically and emotionally demanding, yet also so exciting. Looking down at my enlarged belly, I started to take more notice of every movement: the turns and hiccups, or the feeling of baby lying on my bladder, resulting in frequent trips to the bathroom.

I felt emotional at the thought of meeting my little one, as well as some fear and anxiety surrounding the birth. *How my life is going to change once baby comes along. How will I even know what to do?*

Whenever I started to feel anxious, I practised deep belly-breathing (see opposite), which helped soothe my nerves.
And I tried my best to slow down and enjoy the final weeks with my baby in my tummy, as impatient as I was to meet this little one who would change our lives forever.

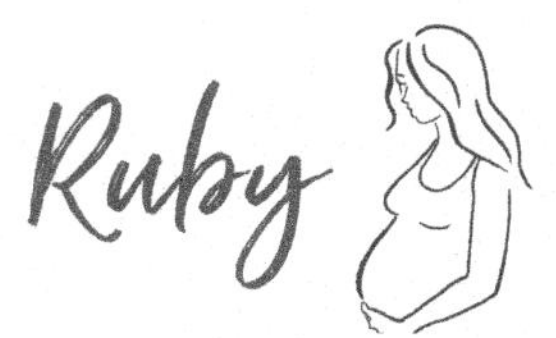

SELF-CARE IN THE THIRD TRIMESTER

It's important to make time to attend to your own needs before baby arrives. Here are some ways to take care of yourself in the final months of pregnancy:

- Nourish your body with healthy food. Aim to eat wholefoods, rather than reaching for something in a packet.
- Forget the countdown: slow down and enjoy the journey. Spend quality time with friends and family. Swim in the ocean or take a walk in nature. Make sure you get plenty of rest.
- Practise deep belly-breathing. You can do this by breathing in for the count of 4, holding for 4 and breathing out for 4. Practising breathing and mindfulness techniques can combat negative thoughts or over-thinking. Deep breathing may also be beneficial for labour and birth, plus it's a wonderful tool for motherhood!
- Don't Google it! I admit I struggled with this one. During my second pregnancy, I decided to stop looking up every question online and instead to wait for my antenatal appointments. As a result, I felt a lot more relaxed.
- Get creative. Paint, draw, colour, knit, sew or write. You might like to make something for your little one's nursery.
- Nest. One of my favourite parts of pregnancy. Preparing the home for your new arrival can be good for the soul. It's also a lovely way to bond with your partner.

And some things your partner can do:

- Talk about the birth plan and discuss what is important to you both.
- Get prepared for the birth in a practical way. Fit the carseat, fill the car with petrol and know the route to hospital.
- Go out for a date night and enjoy time together, just the two of you!

David

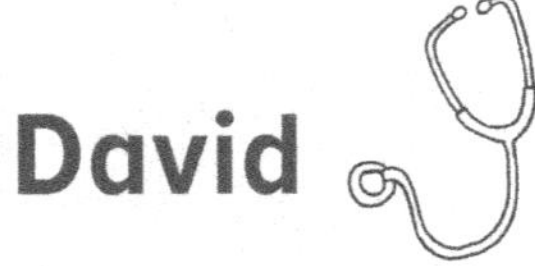

GROUP B STREPTOCOCCUS

Group B streptococcus (GBS) is a bacteria that is commonly found in the gastrointestinal tract of all people and, from time to time, on the skin of the perineum or in the vagina for women. It can come and go and is not generally a problem when it is in these areas in adults. However, GBS can be a cause of disease if it colonises the placenta or amniotic sac. It can also be a cause of severe infection for the newborn baby, leading to a condition called sepsis, which can be life-threatening to a baby. GBS carriage is very common. GBS sepsis is, thankfully, uncommon, but due to its association with cases of newborn deaths and stillbirths, some vigilance is required.

The GBS swab might not be a routine test, depending on which state of Australia you live in, but it is still something that all states (or obstetricians) will have a policy or system in place for screening and/or treating.

There are two main schools of thought when it comes to prevention of GBS-related pregnancy complications. In 'universal screening', all women are offered a screening swab, usually at around 36 weeks, and those returning positive on the swab will be offered antibiotic treatment in labour. In 'risk-based screening', only women carrying babies at increased risk of GBS sepsis are screened and/or treated with antibiotics in labour without screening. Factors used in this assessment include the length of labour, time from broken waters, any prematurity for the baby, infectious signs such as fever or a history of a GBS-affected infant. Both approaches are valid and have their pros and cons.

In my part of Australia, I see women from both sides of the New South Wales and Queensland border. In Queensland, risk-based screening has previously been recommended. In New South Wales, universal screening is more commonly undertaken, though each hospital has the option to make their own policy. I can appreciate the pitfalls of each. With universal screening, a lot of women will be given IV lines and antibiotics for short, uncomplicated labours and in some cases, practitioners may be falsely reassured and hold off antibiotics because of a negative swab. With risk-based screening, we often have to work in the dark about the possibility of carriage and this may lead to earlier intervention in some instances, such as when the waters break before labour begins.

One concern I often have to address with patients is a concern that a positive result will lead to intervention in their birth experience. While couples have the right to make an informed choice about investigation and management of their pregnancy and birth, as with all screening tests, I encourage them not to avoid the test due to a fear of implications, but to use the test result for a proper discussion about the relevance of the result in their particular circumstances.

Most practitioners are happy for women to self-collect a swab for GBS screening. To do it properly, though, it should be from the whole area from which the bacteria could potentially be exposed to the baby. This means the swab should go into the vagina, then across the perineum, then into the anus – a difficult exercise in coordination when you are 36 weeks pregnant.

What does it mean if I am GBS positive?

Firstly, don't worry. As mentioned above, GBS carriage is common and can come and go. A properly collected swab will show up GBS positive in as many as 1 in 4 women. In places that adopt universal screening, this swab is done within a month of the birth because of the fact that it can be transient. Being GBS positive does not make you dirty and does not mean that you have an infection that needs treatment. What it means is that you have a small increase in the possibility of the baby or placenta being colonised by the bacteria after your waters are broken, or when you are in labour.

For this reason, a GBS positive swab has a few implications for recommended safe management of full-term pregnancy. When a woman is known to be carrying GBS in labour, it will usually be suggested that antibiotics are given during active labour, or at least from the point after the waters are broken. This means an IV line will be needed, but it doesn't need to be continually hooked up, and a dose of antibiotics will be given every 4–8 hours during labour, depending on the antibiotic choice.

The other main implication of a positive GBS result is related to a situation where the waters break before any other sign of labour. This is called prelabour rupture of membranes (see page 155). Most obstetricians will take the GBS result into account when helping to advise women about how long to wait for labour after the waters break. In most cases, a positive GBS result will mean that a recommendation will be made to start labour sooner rather than later to avoid the possibility of the bacteria ascending into the uterus. Some practitioners would treat an unknown result (for somebody who declined the test) in the same way. With a negative swab result, there may be some further leeway in waiting longer to induce labour if the waters break before the contractions start.

But what about the good bugs?

Some patients worry that the antibiotics will have a negative effect on the healthy bacteria, which is important for baby to be exposed to in order to establish a normal balance in the intestinal tract and potentially help with immune system development. The antibiotic choice is usually what is called narrow spectrum (and often a type of penicillin, unless you are allergic), which means that it does not knock off all bacteria, but is focused more towards the group B streptococcus. There will also be plenty of time for baby to be exposed to your microbiome after the birth.

Paediatric doctors will usually be interested in the GBS status of the mother, and whether or not antibiotics were given, when they are looking after a baby. Having antibiotics during labour may be taken into account if your baby ends up needing care in the nursery and may sway opinions about length of observation, or whether or not the baby is recommended to be given antibiotics directly, in certain circumstances. For couples who are worried about antibiotic exposure for the baby, a dose or two for the mother during labour can sometimes change recommendations for baby to be given antibiotics directly after birth. If antibiotic exposure around the birth does end up having an impact on you, there are many recommended perinatal and postnatal probiotic products, or natural methods, that can help to re-establish a healthy microbiome.

VACCINATIONS

There are two main vaccines currently recommended for women to get during their pregnancy. One is for influenza, the other is for *Bordetella pertussis* (whooping cough). Neither of these bugs are known to cause birth defects or have major permanent effects on the unborn baby during pregnancy.

Influenza is mainly a concern for pregnant women because they are classified as an at-risk group. In other words, if you are pregnant and happen to get the flu, it is possible that it could make you much sicker than a non-pregnant person. This is partly because the immune system is a little more vulnerable during pregnancy, and partly because the lung capacity is reduced, making chest infections and progression to more serious illness, such as pneumonia, relatively more likely. You can get the flu vaccine at any time during pregnancy, but it is generally best to wait until the yearly updated vaccine is out to get the most benefit. If you do happen to get the flu while pregnant, don't be too concerned. The main things you need to do are keep well hydrated and watch out for any fever. If you do get a fever, treat it early with paracetamol and let your doctor or midwife know.

The whooping cough vaccine is a little different. Adult whooping cough is often not very severe. Newborn infants can become very unwell if they develop severe respiratory infections, particularly whooping cough, due to its more severe effects on their smaller upper airway and larynx. The vaccine is not so much for the pregnant woman as it is for the baby to develop passive immunity. When you are first vaccinated, your immune system makes a smaller type of antibody that is only present for a few months after exposure to the vaccine. The longer-lasting antibodies, which can hang around for years, are differently structured and do not cross the placenta. The early 'acute phase' antibodies for whooping cough are able to cross the placenta and enter baby's bloodstream. This means that when they are born, they will have some pre-existing protection. For this reason, it is currently recommended to get a whooping cough vaccine from 28 weeks of pregnancy, as this will give baby maximum benefit by the time of birth, without wearing off beforehand. This is recommended even if you only recently had the vaccine (as it lasts 7 or so years in adults otherwise). There is no harm in you having an early booster.

COMMON QUESTIONS WITH (USUALLY) EASY ANSWERS

WHAT CAN I DO ABOUT THIS HAEMORRHOID?

Most haemorrhoids will go away within weeks after the birth. Blood has a harder time getting back up towards your heart when you are pregnant, which is why puffy ankles and varicose veins are also a problem for heavily pregnant women. When the baby and placenta are out this pressure reduces, so all of these problems get better.

Haemorrhoids are painful though and can often bleed fresh blood, so are a valid concern. 'Tough it out until the baby is born' does not usually cut it as an answer. Try these measures to treat haemorrhoids:

- Avoid straining due to constipation by increasing dietary fibre or taking low-dose laxative medications, if required.
- Stay well hydrated (this will help keep stools softer).
- Use flushable wet wipes instead of toilet paper to avoid scratching the surface (causing pain and bleeding).
- Most over-the-counter haemorrhoid creams are safe in pregnancy. They usually have a combination of a barrier cream, local anaesthetic or mild steroid in them, all of which are safe in pregnancy. It is worth checking particular products with your doctor before use.

Surgery for haemorrhoids can be safely done in pregnancy, but as most resolve after birth, this is only done in severe cases. I generally reassure women I will happily refer them to have haemorrhoids surgically removed if they are still there a month after the birth.

WHY AM I ITCHY?

Most itches during pregnancy are quite harmless. The most common type of itch is often felt around the centre of the abdomen (around the belly button) and skin over the growing uterus. It can be associated with a red, blotchy rash that comes and goes. This is called PUPPPS, for pruritic urticarial papules and plaques of pregnancy. These are annoying, but harmless – falling into that category of 'pregnancy weirdness' that happens in your body in relation to changes in hormones, your immune system and the person growing inside you who is 50 per cent somebody else.

There are whole books about changes in the skin during pregnancy. Occasionally, there are conditions that respond to steroid creams (most of which are quite safe to use in pregnancy). Women with eczema may find it flares during pregnancy also. The only potentially dangerous condition associated with excessive itchiness is called obstetric cholestasis. This condition is a build-up of something called bile salts, which are produced by the liver and can become excessive during pregnancy in some women. They tend to produce itchiness that is most prominent in the extremities (i.e. the hands and feet). This condition does have a small association with late stillbirth, so it is important to know about. Treatment involves medication and an early induction of labour, after 37 weeks. Thankfully, this condition is quite easily excluded with a blood test, which your doctor will likely request if you are concerned by this type of sudden itch, particularly in the second half of the pregnancy.

Itches that are not caused by obstetric cholestasis can often be treated with an over-the-counter antihistamine medication. A lot of the more modern drugs in this class are category B for pregnancy (not known to be harmful, but also not proven to be safe). Some older drugs for itchiness are category A (thought to be safe), but may also cause drowsiness. Discuss with your doctor before taking these medications.

IS IT SAFE TO SLEEP ON MY BACK?

Try to avoid lying flat on your back in the third trimester. As your uterus grows, it starts to rise up past your belly button and towards your rib cage. It also gets heavier. By 20 weeks, it will usually be around the level of your belly button and by 28 weeks baby will generally be orientated up and down, mostly head first. The major blood vessels going to and from your heart – the aorta and the vena cava – run down the front of your spine, before splitting into two, roughly around the level of your belly button.

The combination of these two things leads to the possibility of the big blood vessels to and from your heart getting squashed. Medically, we call this aortocaval compression. If you are awake and alert, you will become aware if this is happening, because you will suddenly feel very light-headed or nauseous, like you are going to faint.

The most common time in pregnancy that this becomes an issue is if you end up needing an epidural/spinal anaesthetic during labour, or for a caesarean. In these circumstances, low blood pressure and nausea can be issues that we are prepared for. Commonly, women with epidural/spinal anaesthetics are nursed on their side, or with something under their hip and lower back to tilt them slightly to the left, which takes this pressure off the blood vessels. When women are in labour with an epidural, there is generally a continuous heart monitor on the baby for this reason. This compression can sometimes cause the baby to show signs of stress based on the heart pattern, and the monitoring allows us to correct position or blood pressure if this occurs.

An extension from these observations in hospital settings is the question of whether this same thing happens during sleep when women are not in labour. You would expect that a significant change in blood pressure would cause you to wake or come out of deep sleep enough to reposition and take this pressure off – and this is what likely happens in healthy women.

If the compression is minor enough to have an impact on the blood flow to the uterus, but not the blood pressure sensors in your brain, theoretically this may put baby at risk. Other factors involved may include any obesity in the mother, deep sleepers, or women with sleep apnoea. Most scientific studies looking at maternal sleep position are trying to establish a link to stillbirth. Because stillbirth is not a very common thing, it would require a long time and a lot of women to prove this link. Most expert opinion and the evidence from smaller studies seems to point to side-sleeping as being the safest thing to do. However, if you are trying to be a side-sleeper but keep waking up on your back, don't be too alarmed. Look out for the baby's normal movement patterns and talk with your doctor or midwife about sleeping habits in pregnancy to see if there is anything they can do to help.

IS THIS VAGINAL DISCHARGE NORMAL?

Probably. A lot of pregnant women describe increased moisture when they are in the third trimester. The glands in the vagina go into overdrive during pregnancy, getting things extra lubricated for birth. This can result in new dampness, which occasionally takes women by surprise. The medical term for this is leucorrhoea.

As labour draws closer, a thicker mucus 'show' can also be common, and is a good sign that the cervix is getting ready for birth.

It is worth discussing any changes in vaginal secretions during your check-up, because there are some things that can cause an unhealthy discharge. It is also possible your waters can break early and well before labour.

Why is my friend's bump bigger than mine?

Everyone's body is different, just like every baby is different. The fact that your baby bump is smaller or larger than that of a friend doesn't determine anything. We all carry our babies differently; some of us carry low, others have a belly that appears higher. We all gain varied amounts of weight during pregnancy and some hold more body fluid than others. Try not to compare when it comes to the size of your bump.

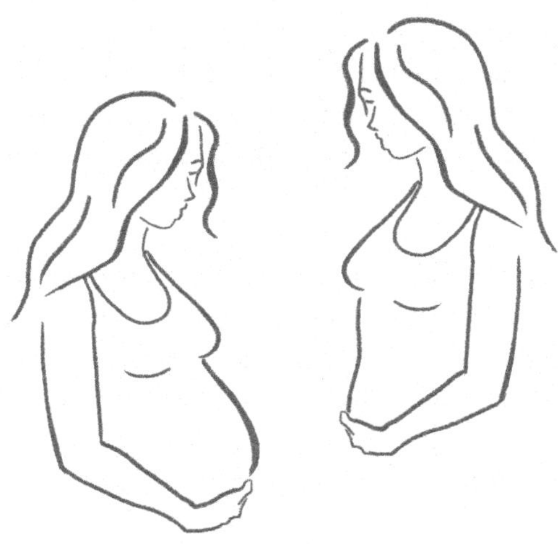

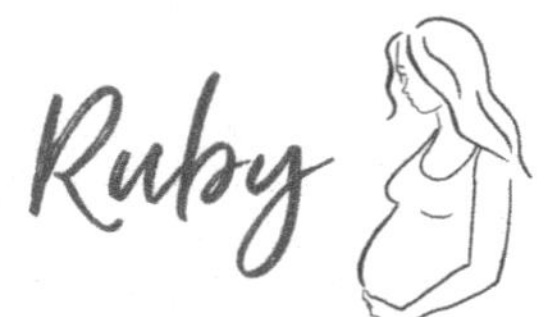

SYMPTOMS AND SIDE EFFECTS

LOWER BACK PAIN

By the end of your pregnancy, there will be 5 kg or so extra weight pushing out in front of you, from your enlarged uterus as well as the fluid and baby inside. Your centre of gravity will have shifted and the muscles of your spine will be working harder to compensate for this. Most women describe lower back discomfort during pregnancy. Occasionally, this becomes more significant, interfering with day-to-day activities or requiring pain medication. Sometimes, a shift in the bones of the lower spine can cause pressure on the nerves going down the legs, known as sciatica.

While uncomfortable, lower back symptoms in pregnancy are rarely dangerous. The main treatment options are heat packs, physiotherapy and pain relief medication if needed (see page 108). Having a massage by a professional can also help. This usually requires lying on your side; however, some massage therapists have special tables that have a hole to accommodate your belly.

Women who have experienced back problems often question whether it is safe to give birth naturally. It is important to discuss your personal details with your doctor, but in most cases natural birth would be recommended. It will probably be advised that you consider a discussion with an anaesthetist prior to labour, though, particularly if you have had surgery on your spine. Some back injuries, or surgeries, may make it more difficult for an epidural anaesthetic to be used.

LEG CRAMPS

Leg cramps are common in the second and third trimesters, especially at night, and usually occur in the calf muscles and feet.

Magnesium is often taken for muscle cramps or restless legs and is safe to use in normal doses. Using magnesium cream is also an option. When cramping occurs, straighten the leg and flex your foot towards you. Stretching or massaging the calf muscles can also be beneficial.

FATIGUE

You may be feeling as though first trimester fatigue is back, and back with a vengeance. This is very common. Your baby is gaining much of their weight in the last few weeks, plus you may be finding it difficult to sleep at night due to discomfort, heartburn or the many trips to the bathroom, all leading to exhaustion. It's important to listen to your body and rest as much as you can, anywhere you can get comfortable – even if this means falling asleep on the sofa or in a chair.

Tips for coping with third trimester fatigue:

- Ask for help (and accept it). If someone offers to cook a meal or carry the groceries, say yes!
- Exercise or get fresh air when you feel most energetic. This tends to be the mornings (although everyone is different).
- Continue to eat well and drink plenty of water to stay hydrated, even if it means more trips to the bathroom.
- Have a massage. Whether it be a pregnancy massage by a trained professional or a foot rub from your partner, this can be a perfect way to ease fatigue at the end of the day.

SWOLLEN FEET

Swollen feet and puffy ankles caused by fluid retention (known as oedema) can be a real nuisance as you near the end of your pregnancy. Swelling can be eased by elevating your feet, and if you work sitting down for most of the day, it's a good idea to get up and walk around regularly to help with blood flow. Stockings are also available, which, although not overly comfortable to wear, are helpful. Note that swelling accompanied by headaches, dizziness or abdominal pain can be a sign of preeclampsia, so it is important to let your doctor know if you have noticed any of these symptoms.

LEAKING BREASTS

Yes, your breasts may begin leaking even before you give birth. This is, in fact, relatively common. If you are worried about leaking in public, you can always invest in cotton breastpads; these will also come in handy if you breastfeed once baby arrives.

CARPAL TUNNEL SYNDROME

Carpal tunnel syndrome is caused by pressure on the median nerve, which may cause a tingling sensation or pins and needles, numbness, pain or swelling in the hand and wrist. It occurs during pregnancy due to the build up and retention of fluid, which can be common in pregnancy. It is often worse at night, and driving, writing or typing can cause discomfort or pain. It usually improves following birth, after a few days or weeks. Alleviate pain by avoiding repetitive movements if possible. Ask for help with carrying heavy objects, such as the food shopping. Your doctor or physiotherapist may recommend a splint if the pain is severe.

BRAXTON HICKS

Braxton Hicks are essentially false labour contractions. This is the uterus preparing for birth. They can begin as early as the first trimester, and tend to be short, painless and nothing to worry about. The sensation is like a tightening in your uterus or across your belly; your stomach can feel hard and tight, and then the feeling subsides. Some women may not experience Braxton Hicks at all throughout their pregnancy, and that is completely okay.

Braxton Hicks are usually irregular and stop once you move or change position. If you're experiencing contractions and are unsure whether they are Braxton Hicks or labour pains, speak to your doctor or midwife, particularly if you are in the later stages of pregnancy. If you feel contractions are becoming stronger, more frequent and closer together, it's best to get in contact with your doctor or midwives at your local hospital.

There isn't a lot you can do when it comes to Braxton Hicks besides wait for them to pass which, in most cases, is quickly. However, there are a few things that may help relax you and alleviate any discomfort:

- Lie down, or find a comfortable position that best works for you.
- Go for a walk or move around.
- Take a warm bath or shower.

PERINEAL MASSAGE

Perineal massage can be done as preparation for vaginal birth. As this is the area where tears are most likely to occur during birth, stretching and massaging the perineum – the skin between your vagina and anus – can reduce the risk of tearing, particularly in first-time mothers. You can start perineal massage from 35 weeks onwards (it is recommended that you do not start it prior to this). Research shows that perineal massage only needs to be done once or twice a week to have benefits.

Perineal massage involves placing either your thumb or two fingers (whatever is most comfortable) into your vagina around 3–5 cm deep, and gently yet firmly applying pressure downwards towards the rectum to stretch the perineum. Stretch the skin downwards and outwards for 1–2 minutes; you will feel a tingling and stretching sensation, however, it should not be painful. The first few times the sensation may be a little more intense but as you do it in the final weeks leading up to birth, this will ease. Practising your breathing and relaxing as you massage is also excellent preparation for birth. If you experience pain or discomfort, discontinue and speak with your doctor or midwife as to why this might be the case.

If you have any pre-existing pregnancy conditions, such as placenta praevia (see page 139), preeclampsia or vaginal infections, it is important to talk with your doctor or midwife to assess whether perineal massage is safe for you.

Tips for perineal massage:

- Take a warm shower beforehand to help you to relax.
- Empty your bladder.
- Ensure you have clean hands.
- You may find it easier to use a mirror, at least at the start.
- Find a quiet, private and comfortable place to sit or lie (propping yourself on pillows can alleviate back pain or discomfort).
- Use a water-based lubricant.
- If you feel comfortable, you may like to ask your partner to assist you.

GETTING READY FOR BABY

When it comes to your first pregnancy, you might be unsure of what practical steps you need to take in preparation for baby's arrival. Getting some things prepared earlier rather than later will help you to relax and stress less leading up to the birth. This may be simply paying bills, planning care for your pet or preparing frozen meals.

NESTING

You might be starting to get the urge to 'nest' as you near your due date. You may be eager to bake, declutter the house or spend a day washing and folding baby clothes. Knowing that everything is organised at home and ready for baby's arrival can allow you to relax and focus on yourself for the last few weeks of pregnancy. Below is a list of tasks that are good to tick off before the birth, to help ease the transition of bringing baby home.

- Have your hospital bag at the ready.
- Install your baby's car seat or capsule.
- Assemble your baby's bassinet or cot.
- Cook loads of meals and freeze them. It sounds tedious, but I promise you will be thanking yourself when you're tired and hungry and there is a home-cooked meal ready to go.
- Create a space for feeding. Make sure you have a comfortable chair and a water bottle, bib or muslin wrap, breastpads and snacks in arm's reach. Sterilise bottles and equipment if you plan on bottle-feeding.
- Stock up on nappies and wipes, plus toilet paper and other essential household items.
- Give the house a clean, even if it is just the floors and bathroom. You will feel relieved coming home to a sparkling house.
- Pay any bills.
- Finalise any paperwork, such as for parental leave.
- Arrange care for your pet or organise a place for them to stay, in case you spend longer than expected in hospital.
- Fill a 'postpartum box' with maternity pads, breastpads, wipes, nail clippers, hair elastics, reading material, snacks etc.

Setting up the nursery

In my mind, there is nothing more therapeutic than creating your baby's nursery in the weeks leading up to bringing them into the world. This is such a special time for both you and your partner, and a way for your partner to connect with their unborn baby. Here are some ideas for setting up the nursery:

- Consider the little things that will help create a space that is organised, peaceful and homely.
- Think about different spaces for changing, sleeping, nursing, etc.
- Always make sure your choice of sleeping arrangement, whether it be bassinet, cot or co-sleeping, is safe. Refer to Red Nose safe sleeping guidelines (see rednose.com.au).
- Many babies love looking at a mobile above the change table.
- You don't need to go out and buy an expensive nursing chair. Choose one that is comfortable, easy to get in and out of (remember you'll be holding the baby when you do!) and will allow you to relax and sit comfortably for a while.

WHAT WILL MY BABY NEED?

Walking around a baby store or searching online for baby products can be overwhelming at first. There seem to be so many 'must-haves', it's hard to work out what is really essential and what you can go without. This checklist contains the key items that are best purchased before baby comes along. You may need additional items, such as a bouncer, baby bath or breast pump, but these can be bought in the weeks following the birth, depending on your specific needs and lifestyle. The Red Nose website provides important and relevant information when it comes to purchasing baby items, particularly if you are thinking of buying second-hand, hiring or borrowing from friends or family.

- Car seat/car capsule – A safe car seat or capsule suitable for a newborn should be installed around week 36 of pregnancy.
- Bassinet or cot – Red Nose recommends your baby sleeps in the same room as you for the first 6–12 months. Newborns can sleep in a cot from birth, but you may choose to have a bassinet at first, then transition baby into his/her own cot when they're older.
- Pram.

- Change table.
- Muslin wraps (for wrapping baby or catching spews).
- First aid kit, including thermometer and baby cotton buds.
- Bodysuits – For a summer baby, sleeveless or short-sleeved; for a winter baby, long-sleeved.
- Baby wraps/sleeping bags.
- Baby wipes.
- Newborn-size nappies.

CLOTH NAPPIES VS DISPOSABLES

CLOTH

Pros:

- Environmentally friendly.
- More affordable in the long-term. The outlay at the beginning may be expensive but they can be reused of course. Some cloth nappies are now one size and can be expanded with press studs or velcro as your child grows.

Cons:

- Be prepared for a lot of extra work: soaking, washing and drying.
- Washing and drying also uses a lot of water and electricity (especially if you are unable to dry them outside due to the weather).
- They are generally less absorbent than disposable nappies.

DISPOSABLES

Pros:

- Practical and easy to use.
- They tend to absorb better than cloth nappies.

Cons:

- Expensive.
- They are single use and end up in landfill.

PACKING THE HOSPITAL BAG

Here is a checklist for you and baby. Keep in mind that if you are having a C-section or expecting twins, your stay may be longer, typically 3–5 nights for a C-section compared with anything from 4 hours to 2 days (longer if there are complications) for vaginal birth.

For mum:

- Medicare card and health insurance information.
- Sleepwear or loungewear – something that is easy to breastfeed in. Choose dark colours, particularly for pants (to help hide any stains).
- Pair of warm socks.
- Several pairs of dark underwear.
- Maternity pads (aka 'surfboard' pads).
- Maternity bras and breastpads.
- Lip balm and nipple cream.

Some little extras:

- Magazines; music; camera/phone (don't forget the chargers); snacks; hand cream and face cream; dry shampoo; your own towel or pillow/pillow case; ear plugs.

For baby:

- Clothing – bodysuits or singlets, depending on the time of year. Make sure they are easy to get on and off with zips or easy-press studs, as tiny babies can be a little difficult to change.
- Newborn-size nappies. Some hospitals only use cloth nappies, so if you prefer to use disposables, make sure you pack some.
- Baby wipes.
- Muslin wraps (5 or more).
- Bottles and formula if you are choosing to bottle-feed.

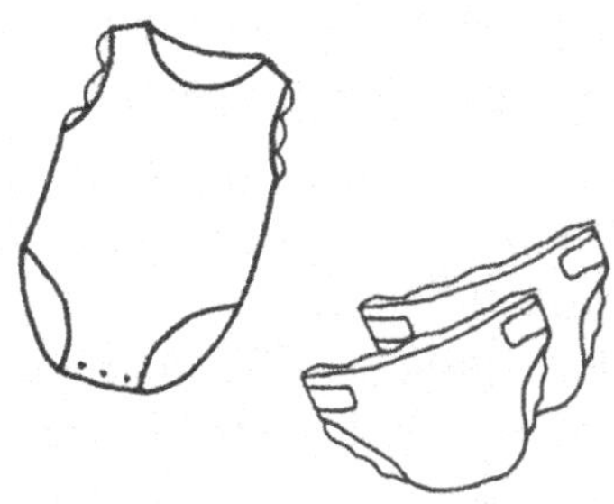

David

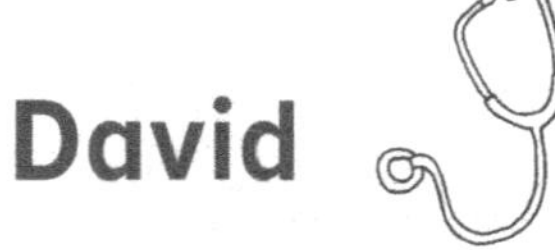

THIRD TRIMESTER SURPRISES

Even as you are hitting your stride with the pregnancy, there are new surprises that may occur in the third trimester. These can be worrying or disappointing, but are often very manageable with the right advice. The following are some of the more common problems.

MY PELVIS FEELS LIKE IT'S GOING TO SPLIT APART!

Some stretching discomfort is very normal during pregnancy. The most common type of stretching pain that women describe is called round ligament pain. These are the supports that run from the top of the uterus into the groin at the top of your pelvis. They often start stretching from the start of the second trimester; this symptom is common between 12–16 weeks.

The uterus is like a hot air balloon, and the bones of the pelvis are the basket at the bottom. As the balloon fills, it starts to tug on the ropes holding it onto the basket. These ropes are your round ligaments. This type of cramping and pain is harmless but can be uncomfortable. If your doctor presses between the bump of your womb and the bony part of your hip, this is the round ligament. The wall of your abdomen can also cause discomfort as it stretches.

Your rectus muscles are long muscles running from under your ribs down to the front of your pubic bone. These are the ones that become a 'six-pack' in people who work out. In pregnant women, these can begin to split in the middle. Usually, this isn't painful but can contribute to cosmetic issues after the baby. It can cause pain and may be linked to a more severe type of pain in the middle of the pubic bones called pubic symphysis diastasis (sometimes called pubic symphysis separation, dysfunction or instability).

Your pelvis is not one bone. It is made up of a ring of bones coming off the base of your spine. The bones are joined by strong bands of fibrous collagen. It is natural for these bands of collagen to stretch a bit during pregnancy. Your placenta will be releasing a lot of hormones to help with this. One particular hormone involved in this process is appropriately named relaxin. This hormone is known to reach peak levels in pregnant women at 14 weeks and also close to delivery. If the collagen gets a little too soft, it can start to cause pain.

Unfortunately, there is no magic cure for pubic symphysis diastasis. Until birth, the mainstays are pain relief, pelvic support girdles and often the advice of a physiotherapist. Most doctors won't support induction of labour until at least 37 weeks for any reason that is not threatening to the baby or mother. Even after the baby is born, it still may take a few months before things completely settle down. Two out of 3 women will have their muscles separate during pregnancy to some degree. Of these women, 3 out of 4 will have the muscles come back together after one year. Very few women may have some ongoing dysfunction of the pelvic bones well after pregnancy. While not painful in itself, it can contribute to other problems with gastric function, spine stability and pelvic floor prolapse. For most women, however, it is a cosmetic concern, and one of the most common things keeping plastic surgeons in business for tummy-tucks.

The biggest risk factors for muscle separation seem to be the number of babies you have and how close together you have them. Caesarean delivery is also a risk factor but may be partially reduced by the surgical technique of the doctor.

I'M BLEEDING

Minor bleeding from the vagina is reasonably common during pregnancy, but you should always tell your doctor or midwife. Most women who experience a fresh bleed in pregnancy find it quite terrifying. Almost always, this blood is your blood, and not that of your baby. The most common reason for minor bleeding is due to normal changes on the tip of the cervix. The glands on your cervix that produce mucous become very active when you are pregnant, and often grow out over the surface in the vagina. These glands have blood vessels close to the surface and can bleed easily when bumped, such as during sex. Having a minor infection, like thrush, may also make you a little more prone to have vaginal bleeding from irritation. A speculum examination can often tell us whether this is the reason for any bleeding. Other things, like polyps on the cervix, can often be found. It will be important for the doctor to know if your pap smears are up to date. Other symptoms involving your bladder or bowel may be significant, such as urinary tract infections or constipation.

If you experience vaginal bleeding, the doctor will want to check:

- That it's not bleeding from under your placenta, which is called an abruption and can be very dangerous for baby.
- Whether it is a sign that your cervix is shortening or opening, which is primarily a problem if you are still preterm.

Abruption – when the placenta starts to come away from the womb

An abruption can be an emergency. If you have active bleeding from the vagina with other signs that baby is under stress, usually indicated by a change in the heart rate, then they will need to be delivered immediately, usually by caesarean. Some minor abruptions can be managed with careful watching, as long as baby shows no signs of stress. Very rarely, bleeding under the placenta can occur without any blood coming out of the vagina, called a concealed abruption. Most women know about these because they cause sudden pain or odd contractions, so while they are 'concealed' emergencies, they are not silent. Be reassured that abruptions are not very common, and most women who experience them have significant risk factors, most commonly relating to unhealthy habits during pregnancy such as smoking or amphetamine use. Chronic medical diseases and higher blood pressure can also contribute to this risk.

Cervical shortening

Heard of the 'bloody show'? It's this blob of mucus and blood that comes out near the end of pregnancy, and is a good sign that your cervix is starting to open up. As the funnel of your cervix flattens and opens, it lets out the mucus plug that had been protecting the baby from the bacteria in the vagina. As it comes out, it often brings a bit of blood from those fragile cervix glands. If this happens near the end of the pregnancy, it can be quite normal. It is definitely still worth telling your doctor or midwife, just in case. This sort of bleeding, close to the due date and with no other symptoms, is a common reason for women to present for unplanned check-ups. Similarly, it can be quite normal to have a few spots of blood after having an internal check of your cervix close to the due date, or a membrane sweep to bring on labour. If you have blood and mucus loss earlier in the pregnancy, it could be a sign that your cervix is shortening and opening prematurely. This can put you at risk of preterm labour and birth.

MY BLOOD PRESSURE IS RISING

Blood pressure is the thing that keeps blood moving about your body. It has a bit to do with how hard and fast your heart beats, as well as how much blood or fluid is in your body, and how open the veins, arteries and tissues are to let blood pass through them. All of this changes a lot throughout pregnancy. For example, by the time a baby is fully grown, one third of a woman's total blood volume is passing through the uterus and placenta every minute. This is a pretty big change from 9 months earlier.

In a normal pregnancy, blood pressure may rise a small amount early on, then it generally falls a bit in the middle, then comes back to normal or a little higher at the end of pregnancy. Generally, if pregnancy is going to cause a problem with high blood pressure, it is in the third trimester. When blood pressure goes up in pregnancy, but everything else is generally okay, this is called gestational hypertension. This is basically an exaggeration of your body's normal response to being heavily pregnant. There are some minor risks associated with having high blood pressure at the end of pregnancy. Sometimes medication might be used to bring blood pressure down. It might also be suggested you have the baby a bit early by induction of labour at the due date or in the week prior. When blood pressure goes up, and it is associated with other particular symptoms or abnormalities on tests, then this can be a more dangerous condition known as preeclampsia.

Preeclampsia

The 'pre' part of preeclampsia is because it comes before eclampsia. Eclampsia is basically having a seizure (a fit) in pregnancy, caused by the pregnancy. Eclampsia is pretty uncommon. Preeclampsia however, is quite common, ranging from mild to severe. It is something that, honestly, nobody really completely understands. It's a bit like having an allergic reaction to your placenta. Just like allergies, we think this condition is at least partially caused by the immune system. Your partner's DNA is the thing you become 'allergic' to at the end of the pregnancy, as the placenta starts to release things into your bloodstream as the due date gets closer. Just like allergies, some people will have only a minor reaction, while some people will have a very dramatic, even life-threatening, reaction.

The type of reaction that a woman has to preeclampsia can be varied. The common things that can happen are as follows:

- The blood vessels spasm. This is what causes the rise in blood pressure. It is most commonly noticed by the patient as a throbbing headache, or as flashing lights in front of the eyes.
- The kidney becomes 'leaky' and starts losing protein into the urine. This is a convenient test for the obstetrician. If it is severe it can cause fluid to collect in the legs (peripheral oedema, otherwise known as cankles), or even onto the lungs, making breathing more difficult.
- The liver can become inflamed. This is not usually noticed by the patient, but occasionally if severe can cause pain under the ribs on the right side of the abdomen. It is usually detected when a blood test shows rising liver enzymes.
- Blood-clotting ability can decrease. This is noticed in a blood test as a fall in the part of blood called platelets. These help form clots, which plug holes in things when they bleed – pretty important when having a baby. The more common annoyance for women is that, if the platelets drop too low, it may be a reason why an anaesthetist will not offer an epidural.
- The nerves can get on edge. This is noticed by the doctor as an increase in reflexes (when they tap under your kneecap, or move your ankle suddenly). The patient may notice a feeling of anxiety or shakiness.
- Preeclampsia can also have an effect on the placenta, which makes it hard for the baby to grow and get enough nutrition. This is called growth restriction or, if severe, placental insufficiency and basically means that the placenta is not working well enough to keep up with the growing baby.

We know that preeclampsia is cured by taking out the placenta, which means delivering the baby too. This is the easy part. The hard part is deciding when to deliver baby, if it happens a bit prematurely in the pregnancy. If you develop preeclampsia before 37 weeks, it becomes a balance between watching carefully to see if the condition progresses quickly and dangerously, versus letting the baby get big enough to do all the things it has to do when born.

Unless it is severe and life-threatening for you or baby, most obstetricians will still aim for a vaginal birth in women with preeclampsia. Interestingly, true preeclamptic women often labour like a champ. It almost seems as if whatever is irritating the nerves and blood vessels has a similar effect on the uterus, which makes it keen to do its thing and get the baby out efficiently.

Most current research seems to suggest the process that will eventually cause preeclampsia starts when the placenta is forming in the first trimester. There are some things that make it more likely to happen to you, such as being your first pregnancy or having twins. There is a lot of research going on regarding ways to stop preeclampsia happening. So far, the most promising treatment is low-dose aspirin started early (before 16 weeks) in women at risk.

After the birth

Preeclampsia can still be a risk for up to 2 weeks after the baby is born. It will usually be recommended that women with preeclampsia be closely watched during this time. If medication has been used before birth to bring the blood pressure down, this may be continued for a number of weeks until things settle down. Even with gestational hypertension, it is still important to watch closely, as preeclampsia can still come on for the first time after birth.

Occasionally, it will be found that women have high blood pressure well after the birth. This usually suggests that they may have had undiagnosed high blood pressure before the pregnancy, or it may be a sign of another medical problem unrelated to the pregnancy.

Most women who have blood pressure problems in pregnancy will make a full recovery. It is important to know that if blood pressure is a problem once in a pregnancy, it is more likely to become a problem in future pregnancies as well. Outright preeclampsia becomes less common with subsequent pregnancies to the same partner, but women who have experienced it before are still more likely to get it again compared to women who have never experienced it.

MY PLACENTA IS TOO LOW

Your uterus is a giant muscle with a funnel on the end. At the top, it is strongest, with the thickest amount of muscle (myometrium) because it has to do all the work of pushing the baby down and out. At the bottom (the cervix) where baby has to come out, the tissue is thinner and stretchier, with progressively less muscle and more collagen or connective tissue. The area where muscle and collagen gradually switch over is called the lower segment. In a normal pregnancy, as the baby gets lower close to your due date, this part of the uterus changes, allowing the baby to get its head into the pelvis (engage) and causing the funnel of the cervix to soften and open up. Your placenta needs to attach to part of your uterus to grow. The placement is, more or less, random as the embryo floats into your womb after conception. Wherever the embryo lands in the womb, that is where your placenta will end up. This is called implantation.

In general, there are four areas where the placenta might develop:

- Anterior: over the front of your womb, closest to your abdominal wall.
- Posterior: at the back of your womb, closest to your spine.
- Fundal: right at the top of your womb.
- Praevia: at the bottom, to some degree over your cervix.

This last position is not a good place for a placenta, as it is obviously the way the baby needs to come out. It is also the least likely place it would go. As the lower part of your womb has much less muscle, it is a less fertile place for your placenta to grow as it seeks a blood supply to nourish the baby.

Most women will not find out where the placenta is developing until the 20-week ultrasound, when it starts to become more obvious. It is reasonably common for radiologists to report low-lying placentas at this stage. Most radiologists will classify a placenta as low-lying if the edge comes within 2 cm of the opening of the cervix. At 20 weeks, your baby weighs only 300–400 g, and your uterus is about a quarter as big as it will be by the end, so things can change in the next 20 weeks. I would say that 9 out of 10 times, a low-lying placenta ends up being well out of the way by the end of the pregnancy, but it definitely needs to be rechecked, usually by about 32–34 weeks, to make sure that it is no longer close to the cervix.

It is common for people to say 'the placenta moved out of the way', but the placenta doesn't sprout legs, shift itself up the womb and lay down roots again. The reason it looks further away by the end is because that lower segment of the uterus is so much stretchier than the upper part, and as it stretches the placenta becomes relatively further from the opening of the cervix.

True placenta praevia is much less common than low-lying placentas, and has much greater implications on your pregnancy and birth. Your placenta is meant to come out last. If it is blocking the exit, there is no safe way for that to happen with a vaginal birth, and you will be advised to have a caesarean birth. The grey zone is if the edge of the placenta is around 2 cm away from your cervix, but not a true praevia. In this circumstance, you will need to have a discussion with the obstetrician about the pros and cons of trialling labour. A big part of this decision may require some patience to wait and see if the head engages, past the edge of the placenta.

Various terms are used to describe placenta praevia, including a grading system, the words 'minor' and 'major', or 'partial' and 'complete'. Most of the relevance of these differences comes down to how the obstetrician will manage the birth and the relative risk of bleeding underneath the placenta. Even delivering baby by caesarean can be a challenging procedure when the placenta is low, especially if it is covering the cervix and the front wall of the uterus. Sometimes the placenta may be delivered first, very quickly followed by baby, or even cut through to get to baby. After the baby is delivered, the area where the placenta implanted around your cervix often has a tendency to bleed, once again because of that lack of muscle in this area.

Most of the time, if you are having a caesarean birth due to placenta praevia, your team will discuss with you the risk of bleeding, including special precautions taken during surgery, the chance of needing donor blood, and the possible interventions required if bleeding becomes excessive and/or difficult to control. Many factors influence the chance of having a major bleed during a caesarean for placenta praevia, so don't be too worried until you have had a discussion with your team about your particular case.

What precautions should I take if my placenta is low?

If you have any bleeding, get seen quickly.

That might seem like stating the obvious, but a little bit of vaginal bleeding in pregnancy can be quite common. There are plenty of harmless reasons why a blood smear might be seen, mostly related to natural changes in the cervix. However, when your placenta is next door neighbour to your cervix, the odds of that blood coming from the placenta are higher. On most occasions, baby will still be fine, but if your placenta is low (especially if it is true praevia), you should not delay being seen if there is any sign of blood. If there are additional signs, like new pain or a change in baby's movements, you should be seen as a matter of highest urgency.

If bleeding keeps on happening, women with placenta praevia may spend long stretches admitted to hospital. This can be frustrating and disruptive to the family, but may be lifesaving for mother and baby if the small bleed ever becomes a massive bleed. When women become long-term residents, many hospitals arrange accommodation near the hospital to try to make things easier, especially if the hospital is far away from home.

Nothing goes in the vagina.

This applies to you, your partner and also your doctor or midwife. If the placenta is known to be low, you may be advised to avoid penetrative sex. This is to avoid 'bumping' the edge of the placenta, which could provoke bleeding. Similarly, doctors and midwives should avoid feeling your cervix with fingertips during any physical examination. Very occasionally, a sterile speculum examination may be necessary, but should be done with the utmost caution by an experienced obstetric doctor. Also, use pads instead of tampons for any bleeding that may occur.

Have some extra monitoring of baby.

A low placenta can sometimes be associated with a small baby, particularly if there has been bleeding or other issues. Having more regular check-ups may be advised, and ultrasound used more frequently in the third trimester to ensure that baby keeps growing, and the placenta is keeping up.

THERE IS TOO MUCH FLUID AROUND MY BABY

This is called polyhydramnios. 'Too much water' would also be an acceptable description. Mums with excessive fluid around baby may have a round, tight tummy (like a beach ball) and find it hard to see strong kicks or feel which bit of baby is where.

Actual polyhydramnios is pretty uncommon. I've seen only a few women carrying around litres and litres of fluid in their tummy, to the point where it is hard to hold up. Most of the time, if the doctor is questioning the amount of fluid around the baby, it is probably just a lot of fluid around a healthy baby. The most widely used way of measuring the fluid around baby is called an amniotic fluid index or AFI. We calculate an AFI by using ultrasound to measure four pockets of fluid (in cm) from each quarter of your uterus.

Having too much fluid around baby means the obstetrician will need to investigate two things:

1. Is there too much fluid because of a problem with baby?
2. Is the amount of fluid around baby likely to cause a problem when the woman goes into labour?

From baby's point of view, fluid is usually a good thing. Most of the fluid around baby is its own urine, so a lot of fluid means a well hydrated baby, in most cases. The fluid is constantly recycled by the baby drinking it. If there is too much fluid, it is important to check that the baby is able to swallow properly (usually by seeing fluid in the stomach on ultrasound). It is also important to check that the baby is not making too much urine. The most common reason for this is because the mother has diabetes in pregnancy, and usually only if the diabetes is not properly controlled by medication. There are also a number of viruses that can impact the amount of fluid around the baby, which can generally be screened for with a blood test.

For the mother, too much fluid means that baby is free to do acrobatics in the womb. This means it is more likely the baby could end up in an odd position when labour starts. It is not unusual for babies to change position from moment to moment when they have a lot of room to move (like they do in the second trimester). When a baby is not reliably in the one position at the end of pregnancy, we call this an unstable lie.

If the waters break during labour and the baby is not in the right position for birth, this usually means a caesarean will be needed. More serious is cord prolapse, in which the baby's umbilical cord drops out of the vagina before the birth.

Doctors tend to dislike leaving things to chance. If your baby is behaving like an acrobat at the end of your pregnancy, then you will be offered more certainty with delivery. Some obstetricians will offer a planned caesarean. This is certainly not the only option for many women, though. It is possible for the baby to be turned head down and then labour induced while baby is pointing in the right direction. If you find yourself with an unstable lie, discuss your options with an obstetrician.

THERE IS NOT ENOUGH FLUID AROUND MY BABY

It is natural for fluid levels around baby to decrease in the last month or so of pregnancy. However, baby still needs a bit of wriggle room and some fluid around the umbilical cord to keep it from getting squashed. If the fluid is low, often the uterus will feel unusually small and tight, and the baby will be less likely to bob back and forth when felt by the doctor or midwife.

If the fluid is a little bit low, it could be totally normal, but your care provider will want to make sure of two things:

1. Have your waters broken?
2. Is your placenta keeping up with the needs of your growing baby?

It is usually quite obvious if you are leaking fluid, but if there is any doubt there are ways for us to test this (see page 154).

If the placenta is not keeping up with baby, this could result in a baby that is not growing, which all midwives and obstetricians are careful to watch for (see opposite). However, if the fluid becomes very low at the end of the pregnancy, the baby is already fully grown, so it is easier to miss a placenta that is wearing out. This is particularly important in women who decide to go more than a week beyond their due date. There are other uncommon reasons for a low amount of fluid around baby, which an obstetrician will take into consideration if they are relevant to a particular pregnancy.

MY BABY IS NOT GROWING (ENOUGH)

Small babies are not necessarily a bad thing. Some women might feel that they are a good thing (easier to push out!). However, there is a difference between a baby that is small because it was destined to be small, and a baby that is small because the placenta couldn't keep up.

The first type of small baby is called 'small for gestational age'. This can be totally normal. There is a range of normal weights at birth. Near the due date, anything between around 2.8 kg to 4.5 kg is normal (or 6 to 9 pounds, for those who insist on using the old measures).

The second type of small baby is referred to as 'growth restricted'. The difference here is usually that the baby had previously been growing normally, but then slowed down or stopped growing for some reason. The rate at which a baby grows is called the growth velocity, and many clinicians will plot weights on a graph so this can be easily appreciated in visual form. With growth restriction, the weight of a baby will be seen to change relative to the average over time. We refer to the size of a baby in centiles, which are basically how the size of your baby compares in a line-up of a hundred babies at the same stage of pregnancy. If a baby starts to fall down the ranks in this line-up, we call it crossing centiles. This is a warning sign that the baby may not be getting what it needs from the placenta.

If the growth of your baby seems to be slowing down, there are a number of things that your care provider can suggest. As most midwives and many obstetricians use a tape measure to estimate the size of the baby, the first step is an ultrasound, which will give a better idea of how big your baby is. To estimate how big your baby is with an ultrasound, measurements are taken from a cross section of the baby's head, abdomen (at the level of the stomach) and the long bone in the thigh (femur), which are then used to estimate of the baby's weight in grams. It is important to be aware that an ultrasound estimate, while probably a bit better than the tape measure, is still an educated guess.

Sometimes the ultrasound report will describe your baby's size in terms of how many weeks along they are. This is confusing because your baby does not change how old they are or when thay are due based on their size at the end of the pregnancy. When an ultrasound report gives a different age in weeks, it is using the average weight and saying that your baby is as big as the average baby would be at that age. Your midwife or doctor will usually be able to clear this up.

In addition to seeing how big the baby is, an ultrasound can also be used to check the fluid around the baby and to look at how easily blood is flowing through the umbilical cord, or sometimes the blood vessels in the baby's brain or close to its heart. These measurements help us to make sure that the placenta is functioning normally and that the baby is not struggling to make blood pass through the placenta and around its body. Even if your baby seems a bit small, if the fluid level and blood flow in the umbilical cord are normal, it can be reassuring that your baby is not in any immediate danger. To tell the difference between a small normal baby and a baby that has stopped growing, we will often need to see if growth changes over time. For this reason, further ultrasounds may be required to keep track of growth if your baby is on the small side.

What does it mean for my labour if my baby is small?

If baby is small, but keeps growing and the placenta is otherwise healthy, there may be nothing that needs to be done other than careful watching and waiting for natural labour. If your baby has slowed down too much, or the placenta shows signs of struggle, then it will likely be suggested that you have your baby early. A baby that is growth-restricted in the womb due to an unhealthy placenta will be better off in the outside world, but of course this depends greatly on how far along you are, as the baby also needs enough time inside the womb so that the organs are fully developed.

After 37 weeks, the decision to deliver a baby that is not growing is easier for the clinician, as concerns about prematurity are mostly over. The decision for an early birth is clearly still a big one. Before 32 weeks in the pregnancy, a decision to deliver due to growth restriction is a much harder one for everybody, as issues of prematurity are much more of a concern before this time and scale dramatically the earlier a baby is born. Before this time, most clinicians would prefer to leave the baby in your womb unless it is absolutely necessary to deliver. Between 32 and 37 weeks is a grey zone, where risk and benefit need to be carefully weighed, but generally speaking, your womb is the best incubator and the preference will be for baby to stay inside as long as possible.

How your baby would be born in the event that growth restriction occurs depends on a lot of factors. All the usual decisions based on your history and health apply. In addition, the obstetrician will look at how significant any issues with the placenta are likely to be, just how small baby is, and how premature the birth will be. Without a good reason to deliver by caesarean, most obstetricians will still aim for a vaginal birth. However, labour does need to be monitored a little more carefully with any suspicion of growth restriction.

When there is any degree of prematurity, you will also need to be prepared for the likelihood that baby will spend some time in the nursery, or intensive care if prematurity is more significant or other factors are involved. As part of decision-making for an early delivery, some hospitals may arrange for you to talk with a paediatrician or neonatologist (baby doctor) before the delivery, and even have a tour of the nursery facilities to familiarise yourself.

If your baby is growth restricted at birth, there is a higher chance this could happen in a future pregnancy. It is a good opportunity to talk with an obstetrician about lifestyle factors that may be modified, or special precautions that can be taken early in a future pregnancy to limit the chances of recurrence. Some common reasons for growth restriction include smoking during pregnancy and preeclampsia.

MY BABY IS TOO BIG

If you are not diabetic during the pregnancy but people are telling you your baby is too big, don't panic. Babies of diabetic mothers can be bigger than average, but they are often disproportionately big due to the higher sugars. Big babies of non-diabetic mothers are often big because that's the way nature intended it (i.e. your genes and your partner's genes), and are more likely to be symmetrically large.

The medical definition of a big baby (macrosomia) is over 4500 g at birth. Some practitioners suggest this is the threshold when an elective caesarean birth should be offered. Research suggests that in non-diabetic mothers, for every couple of thousand women who have a caesarean due to a concern about a baby this size, we only prevent one permanent injury to a baby from an otherwise intended vaginal birth. We call this concept the number needed to treat, and in women with diabetes it is only a couple of hundred caesareans. So caesarean birth for a baby thought to be macrosomic is probably more relevant if you have diabetes. Keep in mind there are complications for women from caesarean birth that are at least as common as the complications that can be caused by a big baby during vaginal birth.

So why worry if my baby is big?

Medically speaking, because of the risk of the baby's shoulders getting stuck after the head comes out (called shoulder dystocia). As I have just explained, though, in non-diabetics this risk is small. If a baby is not going to fit, most of the time we will know about that during labour when . . . the baby doesn't fit. This is called cephalopelvic disproportion (CPD), meaning 'the baby's head is too big for your pelvis'. In the majority of cases, this ends with a caesarean. From the woman's point of view, the fear is that a bigger baby is going to be harder to push out, or cause more tearing. Tearing is far more complicated than just a big head and a small vagina. I have seen 5 kg babies born with the woman needing no stitches, and 2.5 kg babies whose births have caused extensive anal tears. If tearing is a concern for you, talk to your doctor or midwife.

How can I tell if my baby is too big?

You might measure a bit bigger than expected with the tape measure. You also might have had an ultrasound that has told you the baby is bigger than average. Neither of these things is particularly accurate. Ultrasound at full term has a margin of error of almost 1 kg. In other words, if they say your baby is 4 kg, it could reasonably be anywhere between 3.5 kg and 4.5 kg. Similarly, the tape measure is prone to huge variation depending on who does the measuring and their technique, how much body fat you have, how engaged the head of the baby is, and a number of other factors. I freely admit that if I measured twice blindfolded, I would probably get two different measurements. So, use these things as a guide. A few other things could also influence this. One major factor is the amount of fluid around baby, which can often take up as much as 2 litres and make the uterus look and measure larger. If the head isn't engaging in the pelvis around your due date, that can be a sign of a big baby. However, it could also be normal, particularly if it is not your first pregnancy (and you will also probably have a good idea whether this baby feels bigger or smaller than the last). This is the first thing I ask when somebody is seeing me regarding a suspicion of a big baby: 'Do you feel big?' If the woman doesn't feel big, then that is more reassuring than anything.

MY BABY IS NOT MOVING AS MUCH LATELY

NEVER be discouraged from having a check-up if you are concerned about your baby's movements – just go and do it (including right now, if this is the reason you are reading this part of the book).

It is probably okay. This is probably the single most common reason for pregnant women to present for an unplanned check-up with their doctor or midwife, particularly in the last months of the pregnancy.

The concern about decreased movements of the baby is the association with stillbirth. Most women who have experienced a stillbirth describe a decrease in the baby's movements prior to diagnosis. As stillbirth is a relatively uncommon event and can be caused by myriad factors (including many for which we have no explanation), it is not a simple topic.

A large proportion of pregnant women do experience some worry about the movement pattern of their baby. In the past, doctors and midwives would give women kick charts, which they were instructed to vigilantly fill out every time the baby moved, and count to 10 kicks each in 10 episodes of movement per day. This type of arbitrary counting has not been proven to have any true research value in predicting healthy versus at-risk babies. I think it was a way to keep women busy and encourage them to focus on the movements more.

Most women describe the pattern of baby movements changing in the month or two before baby comes out. It is common to describe wriggles or rolls instead of big kicks. There are a few logical explanations for why the movements might change towards the end.

1. Baby is bigger. It has less room for a 'wind up' to a big kick. It is also less likely to be able to perform back flips, or big movements, which are more easily felt by the mother.
2. The amount of fluid around the baby has decreased. This is a natural thing towards the end of the pregnancy and helps encourage the baby to engage its head on the cervix. Less fluid also means less room to move.
3. The head is engaged (hopefully), which some practitioners theorise has an effect on the behaviour of baby due to pressure on the baby's head.

I tell women that the most important thing to be aware of is how often baby moves, and how consistent the baby's normal daily schedule of movement is over time. The outright strength of the kicks is less important, as long as they are present and you can confidently feel them. It is also amazing to see by ultrasound just how active babies can be without the mother feeling a thing, especially if the limbs are pointed inwards towards the spine rather than the mother's skin.

If you are worried, NEVER feel silly having a check-up. Checking a heartbeat and movements takes only a little time and may make you worry a whole lot less.

MY BABY IS UPSIDE DOWN

We all know that babies are usually born head first. Around 1 in 30 babies will not be head down when a woman is at full term. If the baby's bottom is pointing down, it is called breech. This can be very alarming for some patients. A lot of couples will come for discussions with their obstetrician with some negative preconceived ideas about what it means to have a breech birth. But these ideas are unwarranted. Many obstetricians and midwives really enjoy helping a woman through a breech birth.

It can be normal for a baby to be in lots of different positions early in the pregnancy. Most babies will be breech for a period of time. When the baby is still breech at the end of the pregnancy (after 36 weeks), this is called persistent breech. With easy access to ultrasound, it is usually fairly easy to confirm this, but occasionally it comes as a complete surprise to the woman, midwife and obstetrician after labour has already started.

At the end of a pregnancy, the baby is starting to get quite big, and running out of room inside the womb. It is hard for a baby to lie on its side when it is fully grown, so most babies decide to turn to be lying longways inside the womb, called longitudinal lie, and most of the time the baby decides that it is most comfortable to have its head facing downwards, towards the pelvis. There can be some important reasons why the baby decides not to go head down, such as a tight or short cord, an oddly positioned placenta or an unusually shaped womb. Sometimes, the baby may not be head down because of extremes in the amount of fluid around, either not enough making turning difficult, or too much meaning baby has no reason to turn. Most of the time, though, the baby is breech for no concerning reason.

There are three main types of breech position that the baby can be in, and these relate to whether the baby has bent its hips and/or knees. When the baby is coming down with its hips bent, but its knees straight, this is called a frank breech, because when the baby comes out, the first thing that the obstetrician or midwife sees is a pair of buttocks and the baby's genitals. As it comes out, the baby is being frank about its genitals! This is a reasonably common type of breech presentation, where the feet are up around the baby's face, and the baby comes out as if it is folded in half.

When the baby has bent both its knees and its hips, this is called a complete breech. In this position, the baby looks like it is crouching over the pelvis.

When one foot is up, and one foot down, but both hips are flexed, it is called an incomplete breech. This is a little more complicated to manage, but is also the least common way for a baby to lie when it is breech. It is sometimes referred to as a footling breech. A true footling breech is really only something that can happen during labour. The result of this is that one foot can drop into the birth canal before the rest of the baby. This can be a concern because it leaves a gap between the baby's legs where the umbilical cord can slip out, making it difficult for the baby to get blood to and from the placenta.

I'm past 36 weeks and baby is still breech: now what?

Unless the baby turns on its own before labour (which happens very commonly), you have three options:

1. Have an elective caesarean section delivery.
2. Try to have the baby turned to head down, called external cephalic version, or ECV.
3. Give birth to the baby in the breech position.

Elective caesarean

There is nothing wrong with choosing this option if your baby is breech. The reason that elective caesarean birth is offered to women with breech babies at term is because the other two options have some risk associated with them. What it is easy to overlook is that caesarean also has quite a lot of risks – some would argue that it is just as risky as the options of ECV or vaginal breech birth. Caesarean delivery has become such a common way to have a baby that many doctors and patients gloss over the fact that it is still an invasive surgical procedure. The main argument for caesarean birth with breech babies is that it reduces any risk for baby, with the mother accepting more risk for herself. While this is a valid argument in some ways, a caesarean birth does still have some risks for baby.

ECV

External cephalic version refers to having the baby turned by placing external pressure on the woman's uterus. This should generally not be tried until the baby is fully cooked (i.e. over 37 weeks) for two reasons. First, a lot of babies will turn on their own. Second, there is a small chance of any attempt to turn the baby causing some form of distress that would require emergency caesarean delivery, so in such circumstances it is better for the baby to be ready for birth.

The uterus is very soft when it is not in labour, and usually some medication is given to make it even softer. Hands are placed on either side of the baby, one next to the head and one next to the bottom. Pressure is applied directly on the uterus. This changes the way the fluid around the baby is distributed. Slowly but firmly, the hands are moved in either a clockwise or anticlockwise direction (depending on which way the baby is facing). The baby moves to keep in front of the moving pressure on the uterus.

ECV does not always work, though success rates are about 50–60 per cent. Even the best practitioners won't guarantee the baby turning, and it is always better to be prepared to stop rather than risk causing a problem. ECV is generally very safe in the right hands, but does carry about a 1 in 100 risk of complication requiring emergency delivery. This may be due to the cord getting tangled, the waters breaking or the placenta bleeding. If any of these did happen, a caesarean delivery would be performed immediately.

There are a few things that might make the doctor nervous to perform an ECV. These can include a previous caesarean delivery, low fluid, a baby that is too big or too small, or if the cord is around the baby's neck. Not all of these are deal-breakers, though, so a discussion with your doctor can determine if it is still worth a try.

Can I try some natural methods to get my baby to turn to a head-down position?

Although there isn't yet enough research suggesting that any natural methods of trying to turn baby actually work, there are a few things that some women have tried to help get baby to turn. As long as it is safe to do so, you can give these a try:

- Get moving – lying on your side, walking, sitting on an exercise ball.
- Practise pelvic tilts – lie flat and bend your legs with your feet flat on the floor. Raise your pelvis and hips off the ground slowly into a bridge position. Try this pelvic tilt exercise throughout the day.
- Yoga exercises – getting on your hands and knees in a cat–cow yoga pose may help assist baby to move.
- Acupuncture – many women have expressed positive results in baby turning as a result of acupuncture.

Vaginal breech birth

In 2000, the findings of the Term Breech Trial were released. This was a research project in which around 2000 women from across the world who had breech babies after 36 weeks were observed. Half planned to give birth vaginally; half to have an elective caesarean. Among the women who planned to birth vaginally, around 5 per cent of the babies had a serious complication. In the group who planned to have a caesarean, around 2 per cent of the babies had a serious complication. The rate of complications for the women was about the same.

The findings of this study have been debated and reanalysed extensively over the years and there have been many criticisms put forward that seem to suggest breech birth is not as dangerous as the study makes out. One criticism of the study is that the people handling the breech births did not have the same level of expertise, and in some countries had relatively little training in breech birth. Another criticism is that many of the 'bad outcomes' included in the breech group were actually amongst babies that ended up being born by caesarean anyway. This is because the study was 'intention-to-treat' and was based on the way women planned to birth, not the way they actually did.

After the study came out, many hospitals and birthing centres stopped allowing women to try birthing vaginally with a breech baby. The result is that Australia now has two generations of obstetricians: the older obstetricians who used to do breech birth all the time, but for the past 15 years or so only do it every now and then; and the younger obstetricians who trained with a notion that it was a dangerous thing, and often have very limited actual experience with planned breech birth. Thankfully, the tide has been turning a bit over recent years, and many hospitals are starting to offer planned vaginal breech birth again. This means that exposure and confidence with this type of birth is on the rise.

Why is breech birth so different?

In the simplest terms, because the head comes out last. The head is the biggest and least flexible part of a newborn baby. It does have some amazing design features that help it come out, but it is still generally the hardest part to push out. Anybody who has been at a birth knows that once the head is out, the rest of the baby comes out pretty quickly. When the head is the last part to come out though, you can imagine why it is a scary prospect.

One of the major risks for a trapped head during breech birth is with prematurity, because a very premature baby usually has a disproportionately large head, compared with its relatively scrawny body. The woman's cervix also does not have to dilate all the way to let the baby out. The means that the baby's little body can slip through a cervix that is still pretty firm, leaving the head hanging behind.

When a baby comes out breech, the first thing seen is the baby's bottom and genitals. Depending on which type of breech position the baby is in, one or both feet may also be next to the bottom. As the contractions come and the woman pushes, the bottom comes further out followed by the hips, and then the knees. Once the baby's knees are outside of the vagina, usually the legs flex and the little feet drop out as well. Next, the tummy slips down, and at this point, the baby's umbilical cord will begin to be exposed. Once the umbilical cord is out, it is important that the rest of the baby follows fairly quickly. Until the baby is born and able to breathe, it gets all of its oxygen via the umbilical cord. When the umbilical cord is squashed and exposed to air, the blood flow starts to slow down and stop. This means that until the baby has its head out, it is essentially holding its breath.

When the baby is half out, it is very important which way the baby is facing as it comes. For a breech birth, the baby should be facing down towards the mother's bottom, with its back up towards the pubic bone. This is similar to head-first (cephalic) birth, where a posterior birth is much harder if the baby decides to face upwards as it comes out.

There is a common mantra used for teaching breech birth – 'hands off the breech'. Ideally, a straightforward breech birth will happen without you having to do anything. A healthy baby will wriggle and kick as it comes out, almost like it is helping to birth itself. The thought is that if you touch the baby too soon while it is being born, it may become startled and reach out its arms or tense up, interfering with the natural process. However, sometimes a little help may be needed to get the baby out. The key to safely planning to deliver a baby breech is having someone in the room who knows how to step in, and the right time to do it. With the ideal breech birth, all they will need to do is watch.

MY WATERS HAVE BROKEN . . . BUT I'M NOT IN LABOUR

In busy maternity units, almost every day a pregnant patient comes in to have a check-up because they feel their waters may have broken. It is an extremely common concern. A lot of the time, the waters aren't actually broken. There are a number of things in pregnancy that can cause a bit of extra dampness, or a feeling of fluid coming from the vagina. By the end of pregnancy, the glands in the vagina go into overdrive, preparing the body to give birth. Hormones are higher than they have ever been and a lot more blood is pumping down to the vagina, producing extra secretions. This is normal (physiological) discharge that might be different consistency or a larger volume than what you are used to. Medical textbooks give this normal discharge at the end of pregnancy a delightful name – leucorrhoea.

All this extra blood flow, moisture and heat makes the vagina a more hospitable environment for candida (thrush). Internal candida can often cause no irritation symptoms, but can produce a discharge, which can become watery if it is excessive enough. It is very common to get internal thrush in pregnancy. Even women who say they have rarely or never had an issue with candida in the past can find things a bit different in pregnancy. A candida infection is not dangerous to the baby, but some researchers believe it could possibly have an impact on the timing of labour (either early or late) and it can be unpleasant. It is easy to diagnose with a swab, and most internal candida treatments are safe to use throughout pregnancy. Just avoid hard plastic applicators, go for the pessary-shaped options and finish a longer course of 6 nights. It is safer to avoid use of the oral tablets. Other imbalances in the normal microscopic life inhabiting the vagina can also produce watery discharge, but most are harmless to the baby. Another common result is bacterial vaginosis, basically a tipping of the scales from healthy vaginal bacteria to ones that produce a discolouration and odour.

The final thing that can masquerade as broken waters is a bit of bladder weakness. Throughout pregnancy, the baby and uterus put increasing pressure on the bladder. Most pregnant women realise they have to wee more frequently through pregnancy. Some women also can leak a bit with sudden pressure such as coughing, laughing or even standing up too quickly. Occasionally, if the baby is in a funny position, or trying to get its head into the pelvis, a leaking episode may come out of the blue and with no sensation. Urine leakage can be more common in women who have had more babies, and sometimes persists to a degree after the baby is born. A good time to remember to do pelvic floor exercises (see page 96)!

Other times, it is the water from around the baby that is leaking. There are a few tests that can be done quickly and easily to find out if your waters have broken. The first (and easiest) thing to do is to put a pad on. Seeing how quickly a pad becomes wet can give an idea how likely it is to be coming from the uterus. Keep a note of the colour and whether or not the fluid has an unusual odour. If there is a tinge of blood staining (often termed pink liquor), then it is more suggestive of fluid from the cervix or uterus. If it is not obvious, the doctor or midwife may look at the cervix with a speculum to see if fluid can be seen directly coming out. When this is uncertain, there are special swab tests that can be done. Within 15 minutes, these can give a yes or no answer if there is a question of amniotic fluid leaking.

In some cases, an ultrasound done in the office or birth suite can give useful information about how much fluid is around the baby, which can help in decision-making if none of the above provides a clear answer.

What happens after my waters have broken?

You do not have a set amount of fluid for the whole pregnancy. Amniotic fluid is constantly being made, so after your waters have broken, you will continue to have fluid coming away until the baby comes out. Near the due date, more women than not will go into labour within the first 48 hours after the waters break. It is important to keep hydrated, keep an eye out for changes in the colour of the fluid, take your temperature regularly and monitor the normal movements of the baby. If water can come out, bacteria can start to get in, so there is a small chance of rising infection around the placenta and amniotic membranes, which will need discussion with your care providers.

There are some terms you will hear thrown around a bit by doctors and midwives when it comes to broken waters:

- SROM: this is often spoken as 'shromm' and is an abbreviation for 'spontaneous rupture of the membranes'. A woman who has broken her waters is often said to have 'shrommed'.
- PROM: is not the school dance. This stands for, 'pre-labour rupture of the membranes'. It's basically 'shromming' before labour.
- P-PROM: premature prelabour rupture of the membranes, this is shromming before labour, and before you are far enough along in the pregnancy that we would be happy for you to be in labour (i.e. before 37 weeks).

You can SROM in labour all you want, but what if you have PROMmed, or worse still P-PROMmed? What happens then? The answer to this question relies very much on how far along in the pregnancy you are, and is an assessment of the risk of keeping baby inside versus the risk of getting baby out.

Before 34 weeks, it is widely agreed that keeping baby inside is safer than getting baby out. As long as baby is not stressed and there are no signs of infection, most obstetricians will adopt an approach of careful, watchful waiting. Generally, a course of oral antibiotics will be advised, which has been shown in research to improve outcomes for baby and reduce the risk of going into labour too early. It may also be suggested that you be given two injections of a steroid medication called betamethasone. There is more discussion about steroids in the section on premature labour.

Between 34 and 37 weeks, each woman and pregnancy is managed individually based on the feelings of the couple and the obstetrician in the light of any additional factors. In otherwise low-risk pregnancies, this is an area of management that is still debated by obstetricians and researchers as to the best course of action.

After 37 weeks, most clinicians would suggest considering induction of labour. Many hospitals adopt a policy of offering induction of labour within the first 24–48 hours after waters break, when a woman is beyond 37 weeks pregnant. At the end of pregnancy, the cervix is shorter, softer and more open than it is earlier on. Accordingly, the chance of bacteria coming in where it shouldn't be is a little higher, and tends to increase with time from when the waters broke. As baby is pretty much fully cooked at this stage, the decision is more about avoiding this risk of infection balanced against any difficulties or patient feelings towards inducing labour. An important factor in this decision relates to group B streptococcus, which has the highest risk of causing dangerous infections around baby and placenta (see page 116). If a woman is positive for carriage of this bacteria in the vagina, and has broken waters near her due date, most clinicians would recommend induction of labour at the next safe opportunity. Many women elect to go beyond 48 hours with broken waters to allow labour to start of its own accord. This is not reckless, but should involve a discussion with an obstetrician regarding any risks and benefits for their particular pregnancy.

I THINK I AM GOING INTO LABOUR – BUT IT'S TOO EARLY

Signs of labour before your due date (or what doctors call threatened preterm labour) are one of the most common reasons we see pregnant women for unplanned visits at the hospital. Thankfully, a lot of these are false alarms, but certainly some women do go into labour well before their due date, and some of these will be too early to be safe.

Thirty-seven weeks of pregnancy is generally regarded as 'term' for your baby. Going into labour after this is normal and, with an otherwise healthy pregnancy, it just means your baby is ready to come. Just like different women have different lengths of their menstrual cycle, for some women a shorter pregnancy (or a longer pregnancy) can be a variation of normal. Forty weeks is more like an average.

It is common to feel uncomfortable contractions of the uterus prior to full term. If this happens a lot, it's called an irritable uterus. The uterus is a giant muscle, and it can be prone to spasm if something nearby is irritating it. This could be a bladder infection, an upset bowel, stretching of scar tissue or other inflammatory conditions, such as endometriosis. The difference between an irritable uterus and one that is actually going to start true labour can often be hard to tell. By definition, if the cervix is changing or opening, then it is labour. The trick is knowing this might happen before it actually does.

What can be done to see if I'm at risk of preterm labour?

The first step is determining how likely it is that you are in true labour. A midwife or doctor sitting with you and feeling your abdomen will be able to get an idea if the tightenings feel like labour contractions, and also how often they come, how long they last and if they are in a regular pattern. A machine called a cardiotocograph will often be used, both to hear the heartbeat of the baby and detect contractions. If a woman is experiencing preterm contractions, there are two main tests that can be done to determine how likely she is to have preterm birth: fetal fibronectin and ultrasound cervical length.

Fetal fibronectin is the name of a protein found between the wall of the uterus and the bag of waters around the baby. Prior to full term, it should only be detectable in the vagina in very small amounts. If it is found in larger amounts, then the risk of preterm birth occurring is much higher. It is quite easy to test for fetal fibronectin with a vaginal swab test, and a result is available within 20 minutes.

Cervical ultrasound helps to determine risk of preterm birth more commonly in women who are not experiencing labour pains but have other risk factors for preterm birth (particularly a history of it happening previously, or surgery on their cervix). Before the cervix starts dilating in labour, it starts to shorten from the inside out (effacement or funnelling). Changes on the inside part of the cervix (closer to baby than the vagina) can more accurately be assessed with ultrasound than by looking with a speculum. Sometimes, this may even require a long thin ultrasound device being used inside the vagina.

As a general rule, any measurement longer than 2.5 cm is reasonably low risk for preterm birth, but this needs to be taken in context of the starting length of the cervix, how premature the pregnancy is and other factors specific to the woman and her particular experience.

Can premature birth be stopped?

Sort of. . . or, at least, delayed. If a baby is determined to come early, it will usually happen no matter what we do. There are medications that can be given to stop the uterus contracting. These are called tocolytics. One of the most common tablets used in Australian hospitals for delaying preterm labour is nifedipine. These medications are not typically used for long periods of time, but are useful to hold off a preterm birth for up to 48 hours, to allow transfer to a bigger hospital equipped for preterm babies, or to give time for other medications to take effect.

The most beneficial medication for prematurity, from baby's point of view, are steroid injections. The most commonly used steroid injection for prematurity in Australia is a drug called betamethasone. Steroid injections act as a metabolic warning signal for the baby. It is like a hormonal wake-up call for the baby, helping it fast-track some of the systems needed to survive outside the womb, particularly breathing and a substance called surfactant, which is needed for the lungs to expand.

Steroid injections usually come as a pair of shots, 24 hours apart. They have the most benefit for baby if they can be given 48 hours before birth occurs, and this benefit lasts for a bit more than a week before it starts to fade.

It is widely accepted that a single course of steroids given in prematurity has no negative impacts for the baby; indeed many studies since the 1970s have demonstrated the benefits. Giving steroid injections multiple times during a pregnancy is more controversial, so timing this intervention is important.

What will happen if my baby does come early?

Premature birth is a long and complicated issue. Make sure you speak with your obstetrician and, if possible, a neonatologist about your particular case. Before 37 weeks, prematurity becomes a question of how much help the baby will need to do the things it needs to survive in the world, such as breathing, eating and maintaining a normal body temperature. Between 32 and 37 weeks, most babies will need some support and observation regarding these normal functions. They are very unlikely to need a ventilator (breathing support machine) but may need extra oxygen or temporary assistance with the higher pressure in their airway. They will usually be able to attempt attachment to the breast for nutrition, but usually have less energy reserves in their body fat and liver. They are more likely to need supplementation with formula or, if the suck reflex is not fully developed, they may need a tube through the nose into the stomach to directly deliver milk. Most of these babies will do very well in the long term and are less vulnerable to nursery complications or any long-term effects.

Before 32 weeks, babies are likely to need a higher level of observation and care. Most of these babies will be observed in a neonatal intensive care unit (NICU), rather than a general nursery. They are much more likely to need a tube in the throat to assist with breathing (temporarily) and a tube into the stomach to assist with feeding. Handling of babies with this degree of prematurity is more restricted, and they need to be very closely observed because of increased vulnerability to infections and other complications of early premature life.

Very broadly speaking, between 28 and 32 weeks, most babies will do reasonably well in the long run, but it is a very long road, and the risk of complications is higher. Most neonatal units in Australia will only accept care for babies after 24 completed weeks of pregnancy. Before 24 weeks, the odds of a baby surviving, with even the very best of care and technology, are very low, and the odds of permanent disability are high. Between 24 and 28 weeks, there is a gradual improvement in the odds of baby both surviving birth and surviving without long-term physical or intellectual disability. It is very important that any family expecting a baby born in the month or so after 24 weeks be as prepared as possible and speak with all the professionals around them about what can be expected in their particular circumstances.

I AM MORE THAN A WEEK OVERDUE

Basically, you have two options. You can keep waiting, or you can have an induction of labour (see page 176). In most Australian hospitals, an induced labour will be offered if you are more than a week overdue. The magic number in most Australian hospitals is 10. 'Term plus ten' or '40+10' are commonly used phrases when asking why a woman is being induced into labour. What makes 10 special? The baby does not self-destruct after 10 days. There is no 'best before' date printed on your womb.

After 1 week overdue, there are no differences in rates of complications for mother and baby. At 2 weeks' overdue, there does seem to be a small increased risk of complications. We split the difference by starting an induction at 10 days overdue, with the hope that the baby will be out before that time. Many hospitals will have a policy of offered induction after 1 week overdue, while many birth centres will suggest a discussion around induction after 2 weeks.

It is not reckless to wait longer, but it is a controlled risk. The rates of unexplained stillbirth do start to rise after the first week overdue. At term, this risk is around 1 in 1000. At 2 weeks overdue, this risk is 2–3 in 1000, and increases further with time. Now, you could be alarmist and say: 'The risk of your baby dying doubles every week you are overdue!' Or you could be more reassuring and say: 'Statistically, you have an added risk of 1 in 1000 of stillbirth by waiting more than 2 weeks for labour.'

Another issue that can occur due to being overdue is a reduction in the amount of fluid around baby. The baby is also more likely to have passed meconium inside the waters, which can have an impact on the way the birth is managed. Babies do continue to grow after their due date, but the rate of growth is much smaller compared with earlier in the third trimester. Overdue babies are, on average, bigger than term babies, but not dramatically so.

The most overlooked reason to consider an induction by 2 weeks overdue is that it increases your chances of a vaginal delivery. There is increasing evidence that prolonged pregnancy is associated with caesarean delivery. This is a difficult area to study because removing 'operator bias' is so difficult. On the one hand, whatever reason was stopping baby from coming on time is probably going to have an impact on labour and delivery, such as baby not engaging its head early or being in a posterior position. On the other hand, natural factors involved in prolonged gestation, like low fluid or meconium, are more likely to influence care providers in their concern for baby's wellbeing during labour. For example, low fluid pregnancies can make it harder to induce labour and if meconium is present, the use of an oxytocin infusion may be more restrained.

The overall balance of evidence does seem to support earlier induction after term leading to higher success with vaginal birth. In studies looking at induced labour even earlier – at the due date, or in the week or two before, for other medical reasons – there does not seem to be any increased risk of caesarean birth. Some studies even show a decreased risk of vacuum or forceps delivery. There are obviously other factors that determine a successful birth, including the woman's sense of satisfaction with the experience and her perception of pain or interference. All of this will need to be balanced when making a decision. However, I would like to dispel the myth that induction leads to caesarean.

For some women and families, letting labour happen naturally is very important. I find it funny when junior doctors are alarmed if a patient is 'term plus 13' and want to get the baby out immediately, as if those 3 extra days make all the difference in the last 9 months! All risks with pregnancy and childbirth need to be acknowledged, but they should also be treated with respect to the greater picture of the woman's birth. If a woman wants to continue her pregnancy a bit longer than what the doctor and team are comfortable with, extra check-ups or ultrasounds for baby will usually be offered to keep a close eye on things and for added reassurance (for the doctor as well as the patient).

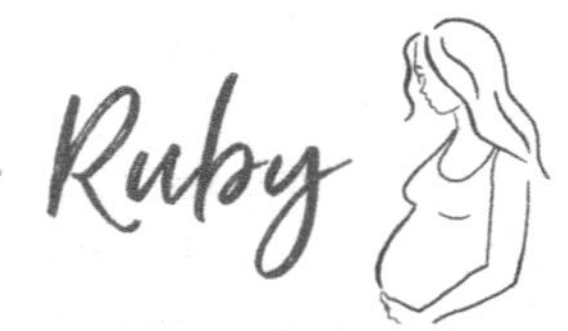

PREPARING FOR THE BIRTH

This is it! Everything leads to this. The nursery is ready, the bags are packed, you've written and rewritten the birth plan, and all you can do now is wait. You may be starting to feel nervous, excited, cautious and impatient, all of which are normal parts of the pregnancy process. It is important to not place expectations on yourself when it comes to the type of birth you want. Just like pregnancy, every birth is unique, and sometimes it may not go as you may have 'planned'. Keeping an open mind, preparing for birth (as much as you can), being realistic in your expectations and positive, knowing that the health and wellbeing of you and your baby is paramount – all of these may help ease disappointment if your birth doesn't go as you hoped. Speaking with your midwives and partner if you are feeling fearful prior to birth is also important, so that they can support you. Remember: there is no failing when it comes to birth.

Sometimes it feels like birth stories all seem to be negative – we rarely hear the positive stories. But they do exist! You may like to seek out more joyful experiences, asking midwives and friends for reassuring birth stories they can share with you. You can also listen to podcasts and read up on positive birth experiences.

Writing a birth plan allows you to communicate to your doctor and/or midwife what you (and your partner) would like to happen during and straight after your baby's birth. A birth plan often includes details about where and how you would like to give birth; the name/s of your support person/people; your preferences for managing pain, monitoring baby, cutting the cord and what happens to your placenta; and any other information you wish to communicate to your birth team. Writing a birth plan is important and empowering, but try not to be too rigid in your expectations; being flexible will help you adjust if things take an unexpected turn.

David

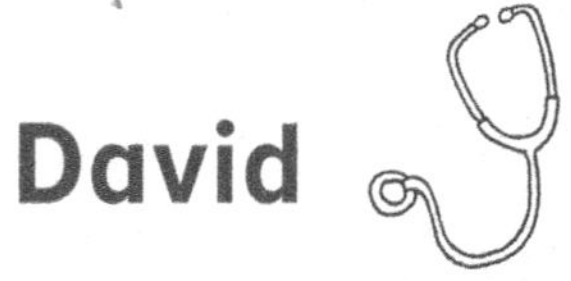

YOUR BIRTH PLAN

There are two very important things to be aware of:

1. Things often change when you are actually in labour (especially your first).
2. Nobody can predict all things, only be prepared for most things.

A good birth plan should be considered more like 'birth preferences'. An ideal birth plan lists all the things you would like to happen, as well as ways to manage the things that you hope don't happen.

A lot of birth plans reference ways to maintain calm, autonomy and dignity during birth, which is great. A birth plan that absolutely excludes all forms of medical intervention may be a little too idealistic and, if strictly followed, may be risky for you or baby.

Try to avoid too many absolutes. For example, 'I have no pain, I don't tear, baby is perfect, I go home in 2 hours' is a great plan. It might happen! But if it doesn't, you may not be prepared for what does happen. One of the biggest dangers of an unrealistic birth plan is disappointment.

A good birth plan discusses things like tearing, operative birth, augmentation of labour and monitoring of the baby. It is important to have some idea about how you might feel if medical intervention is needed at any point, and to use a birth plan as a starting point for a discussion about any worries with your doctor or midwife.

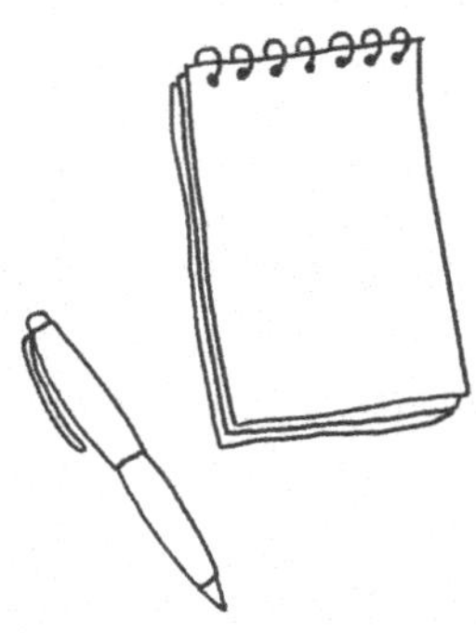

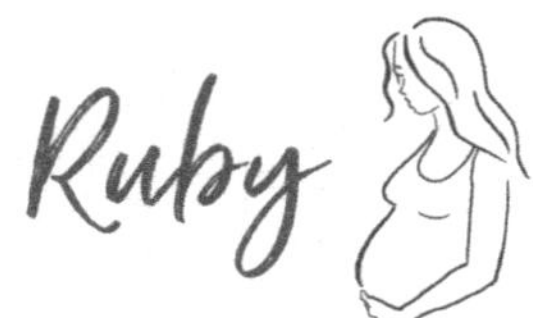

CHOOSING YOUR SUPPORT PERSON

Your support person is a very personal choice. They can be your partner of course; also, if you choose, a family member such as your mother, mother-in-law, sibling or close friend. Some women choose to have a doula, a dedicated support person for birth. Unlike midwives, doulas do not usually have a medical background; they are more focused on helping the woman, both emotionally and physically, throughout the labour and birth.

Birth can be an emotional, challenging and sacred experience, so trust your instincts and choose the person who is right for you. Think about who makes you feel most comfortable, safe and at ease.

Many people struggle seeing their partner in pain, but the midwives are there to support you both through the experience. I will be forever grateful to my midwives for their guidance, knowledge and compassion.

How to tell your mother/mother-in-law/anyone else that you don't want them in the delivery room

Birthing is a very personal, intimate and profound experience. It is hard to predict how it will evolve and how you will feel. So it is always okay to say no to people you may not want in the delivery room, for whatever reason. It is crucial that you communicate your decision about who you may or may not want there – and not feel an ounce of guilt because of it. Be open and honest about your feelings, and ask your family to respect your wishes.

This is your experience, and you get to choose how you make it the best one possible for you. Discuss with your partner whether you will let family and/or friends know when you are in labour, or just share the news once your baby is born. Pencil in a date, whether it be while you are in hospital or when you take baby home, for family and friends to come and visit, but feel able to change your plans!

FEELING ANXIOUS ABOUT CHILDBIRTH

If you are starting to have fears surrounding childbirth as the ninth month closes in, you are not alone. It is important to voice any concerns with your doctor or midwife. It can be beneficial to discuss any fears you are feeling with your partner and close friends and family members too, as they may have some advice or can simply just reassure you.

Worries surrounding childbirth may be about fearing the unknown, or you might be anxious because you've heard stories about difficult births. You might be feeling worried about how you will handle the pain and unsure about pain relief options. Or you may be concerned about the changes that will occur within your relationship after giving birth.

Some things that may assist in easing these fears:

- Talk to those around you who have had positive experiences.
- Be open and honest with your doctor, midwives or doula about your fears.
- Find extra support, or take an antenatal class, to gain more insight into birth.
- Understand that doctors and midwives have heard everything you can imagine, so there is almost nothing they haven't seen before!
- Take a Calm birthing class (see page 172).
- Learn to meditate and practise breathing exercises.
- Create a realistic birth plan, with choices that sit right with you.
- Establish relationships with the health professionals around you so that you feel respected, calm and supported through the entire process.

What if I don't love my baby when she/he is born?

You often hear parents talk about the first moment they held their baby, and the immense and overwhelming love they felt. Many pregnant women (and their partners) worry that they won't experience these feelings.

Your baby is, in fact, designed to help you fall in love with them. Give yourself time to get to know each other without pressures and expectations. Take comfort in knowing that you are both learning. If you don't feel that bond immediately, try to focus instead on enjoying the moment and allow things to develop at their own pace. But it is important to ask for help if you need it.

Midwives often recommend skin-to-skin contact in the early days to help with breastfeeding and settling your baby. Both you and your baby will be undressed as you breastfeed or soothe him/her to sleep. This also encourages the letdown when breastfeeding. From my experience, I believe this gives you confidence, as well as creating a strong bond between you and your baby.

What I'm really thinking:

The final weeks

In the weeks before my due date, I dreamt about birth almost every night. The dreams were vivid and anxious, and I started to fear the prospect of giving birth. I would look down at my huge belly and think: '*I am not ready for this!*' If I could have chosen, I probably would have stayed pregnant for another 9 months!

As you near your own due date, you may be experiencing similar feelings or maybe you're confident, ready and raring to go. Or perhaps your emotions change from day to day, or hour to hour! This is all perfectly normal. Throw in sleepless nights and carrying around all that extra weight, and it's really no surprise this can be an exhausting time, both physically and emotionally. Don't forget about self-care – this is the perfect time to be kind to yourself.

COMMON QUESTIONS AND ANSWERS ABOUT BIRTH

Do I have to be naked?

No. The most important thing is that you feel comfortable throughout your labour and birth. You will most likely be given a gown to wear in hospital; however, you can continue to wear your bra or crop underneath if you feel most comfortable that way. You will want to remove your underwear as it is important that midwives can monitor baby and check your progress at intervals throughout your labour. Or you may feel like having no clothes on at all – and that's absolutely fine too.

What positions are most comfortable?

Every woman and every birth is different. There are a variety of positions you can try – you might like to sit on a birthing ball, kneel, walk around, stand in the shower or recline in the bath. Find the one that feels most comfortable for you.

How can my partner support me during the birth?

Your partner can provide support throughout the birth in a number of different ways, including:

- Giving you verbal reassurance: positive phrases such as 'You're doing so well' or 'You are doing a wonderful job' can be encouraging. (Or you may prefer silence!)
- Supporting you physically during contractions, allowing you to stand yet have your weight supported.
- Giving you a massage on your lower back or shoulders where you might be experiencing discomfort.
- Just being there when you are feeling exhausted by the waves of pain. Simply being by your side may provide you with all the support and reassurance you need.

David

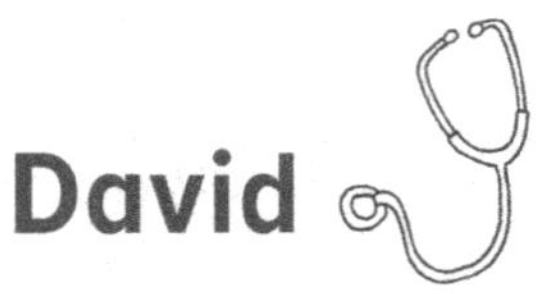

WATER BIRTH

Many birth centres and mainstream hospital birth suites have birthing pools available. While a lot of women choose to get in the pool to deal with the intensity of their labour, many women also choose to birth in the pool. Birthing underwater has been controversial in the past but is gaining a lot of mainstream support when offered in a safe and controlled way. It is important for any woman considering water birth to have a discussion with a professional to explore how suitable this option is for them personally. To help with this, here is a list of some general pros and cons that are applicable in all cases:

Pros

- Water immersion helps a lot of women deal with pain.
- Buoyancy takes the weight off the uterus and abdomen, which may reduce pain and discomfort.
- Body-temperature water may help the muscles around the vagina to relax and soften during pushing.
- Hydrostatic pressure from the water in the pool can support the perineum and may help reduce tearing.
- It is very 'hands off' for the woman.

Cons

- There is an added risk for baby of fresh water aspiration, which could increase the need for breathing support after birth.
- It can be awkward getting out of the bath during an emergency.
- A short umbilical cord (which is unpredictable) can make it hard to bring the baby up out of the water after birth and, on occasion, can result in a snapped cord or other poor outcome.
- It is very 'hands off' for the doctor or midwife, which could be a problem if the head is birthing too quickly (increasing tearing risk), or if help with the shoulders is needed.
- It can sometimes be more difficult to listen to the baby's heartbeat.

It can be alarming to see a baby born underwater the first time, because seeing a baby's head come out underwater, your natural instinct is to bring it to the surface and let it breathe. In principle, it is okay to resist this urge, as until the baby takes its first breath, it is still receiving oxygen through the umbilical cord. It can be normal for a few minutes to pass between the head being born and the baby coming up to the surface. However, even though the baby doesn't necessarily need to breathe in order to get oxygen at this stage, if it starts to attempt breathing before it is out, it can bring water into its lungs. Water does not have the same salt concentration as the amniotic fluid, which is normally in the baby's lungs in the womb. This can cause transient damage and make it harder for the baby to breathe air when it comes to the surface. For this reason, we definitely want babies out of the water before they show any attempt at trying to breathe.

To help prevent the baby's breathing reflex kicking in, we must avoid two things: 1) touching the baby before it is completely born, and 2) a sudden change in temperature or air on the baby's face. This means that a woman birthing in the water needs to stay in the water. If the head is crowning or out, it is either completely underwater or completely outside, no bobbing on the surface. Similarly, if the doctor or midwife needs to go 'hands on' to get the baby out, the water should be immediately drained, or the woman brought out of the bath. Sometimes, we may reach in to help catch a baby that has already been born, but we shouldn't be touching the baby before.

The last thing to remember about getting in the birthing pool is to respect the opinion of the midwife or doctor if they tell you that it is safer to be out of the pool at any time.

Some common reasons why we may recommend staying out of the water include:

- Suspicious changes in the baby's heart rate pattern.
- A change in the colour of the fluid, most importantly meconium, or an abnormal amount of bleeding.
- If the mother develops a fever, or any suspicion of infection exists.
- If it is taking an unusually long time to push baby out, or there is a concern that delivery of the shoulders could be difficult.

Other reasons vary from place to place, but there may also be restrictions based on your weight, or other pre-existing factors. I have had experience with water-birthing mothers who are undergoing induced labour (including on an oxytocin drip), or need a continuous heart monitor for baby. It is not possible to have a water birth with an epidural, and you should not get into water if you have had some particular medications, such as morphine, pethidine or sedatives.

Partners are very welcome to be in the pool for support, or to help catch the baby when it is out. All midwives and obstetricians are very comfortable around nudity when it comes to women in labour, but less so when it comes to the partners, so bathing suits are advisable.

COMMON QUESTIONS ABOUT WATER BIRTH

How will I know when to get in the pool?

Your midwives will begin setting up the birthing pool and prompt you when they feel it is the right time to hop in. Avoid getting in too early, as water immersion can slow down early labour.

How can I maintain my privacy?

You can wear a bikini top, bra or crop top. You may have other requests, such as music and dimmed lighting, which may be worth discussing with your midwife or doctor in the weeks prior.

What happens if I open my bowels?

It is common to open your bowels during birth and this can happen while in the birthing pool. Midwives have seen it ALL before and they will swiftly clean it up. Opening your bowels in the pool may introduce the risk of infection; however, it doesn't mean you will automatically have to get out of the pool. Pools are cleaned thoroughly after use.

If I choose to have a water birth but have a change of mind, is that okay?

Absolutely. Just because you have planned to have a water birth doesn't mean this is what you have to go ahead with. Changing your mind, even in the pool, is okay. You can get out at any point, especially if you decide you want an epidural. Remember, birth plans can change so trust your instincts and do what makes you feel most comfortable.

PAIN RELIEF IN LABOUR

Is labour going to hurt? Short answer: probably.

A lot of midwives and doulas avoid the use of the word 'pain' when it comes to childbirth, referring to labour contractions as 'intensity', 'waves', or 'surges' to avoid colouring the patient's view with the concept of pain. Whatever you want to call it, for most women labour is an endurance sport and very rarely described in any way that could be called comfortable. For simplicity, I will use the word pain to describe a negative feeling towards contractions or birthing.

When it comes to options for dealing with pain there is a basic division – drugs or no drugs. No drugs doesn't necessarily mean 'just deal with it'. While you don't get a medal for getting through without medical pain relief, there are benefits beyond personal satisfaction.

DRUG-FREE OPTIONS

Water – Often when I visit patients during their labour, they are in the shower or the pool. The feeling of water on the skin seems to be a very good distraction from the pain of labour. Temperature is important, as increased sensory input from the skin can help dull the pain response. It is important to stay close to body temperature – no scalding showers or icy baths – as this may have an impact on baby's tolerance of labour or your overall body temperature.

Massage and pressure points – These provide an excellent task for the partner to keep them feeling useful. If you are lucky enough to have a support person who has some alternative-medicine knowledge, they may be able to identify and make use of pressure points to help with pain distraction. One extension of this principle is the use of a TENS machine to directly stimulate nerves and block the pain signal. Some practitioners use sterile water injected under the skin for a similar effect, which can be effective for lower back pain, particularly as the baby's head engages in labour.

Breathing/relaxation – This is all about having your head in the right space for birth and labour. Pain is only what your mind interprets it to be. Calm birthing, hypnobirthing or birth meditation are all centred around the principles of mental preparedness and your ability to detach the negative perception from the physical sensations you have during labour and birth.

The environment – I have grouped some quite important things together here. It is well recognised that pain responses are hugely variable depending on the patient's level of anxiety and fear about what is going on around them. When you are worried, anxious or fearful, your nerves are on edge, ready for a 'fight or flight' response. Your muscles are more tense, and you are hyper-alert. All of this contributes to a heightened sense of pain. Everybody is different when it comes to what makes them calm. Background music, or other calming sound, can be useful. Some people prefer quiet. A lot of women like to avoid artificial lighting, or keep the room dim. I have even done one very memorable birth in pitch blackness – using only a weak pen-light to check with each push if the head was crowning. Vaporisers for aromatherapy are often used as well. Most Australian hospitals will not allow an open flame in medical environments, so candlelight or incense burners are out if you are at the hospital.

What are some natural ways of relaxing during labour?

- Listening to a music playlist that relaxes you.
- Breathing in essential oils.
- Massage.
- Hypnotherapy and visualisation.
- Meditation.
- Positive thinking and affirmations.
- Using a warm compress.
- Deep breathing through your belly.

Hypnobirthing

Hypnobirthing and Calm birthing classes are privately offered antenatal classes that teach women techniques and methods that can help them experience a calmer birth experience. These include breathing techniques, relaxation, self-hypnosis and meditation practices that encourage women to be more at ease and confident going into and throughout labour. Classes also educate partners or support persons on how to encourage these techniques during the birth. Note that these forms of antenatal classes are different to those offered through the hospital or public health system and will usually incur a fee.

DRUGS

Tablets – Paracetamol and codeine are commonly used to help women get through the early stages of labour. Codeine can be habit forming if used frequently for a long time, but a few doses in labour will not cause the baby to go through any drug withdrawal. Most oral tablets will not be strong enough to deal with the peak of labour pain intensity. They are useful leading up to true labour, though. It is important to get some sleep and keep up your energy for the hardest part, so I usually encourage women to use paracetamol, codeine and sometimes a sleeping tablet, to get through the early stages.

Nitrous oxide gas – Also known as 'laughing gas', this is a short-acting pain reliever that requires you to breathe the gas for the duration of the pain. It is out of your system pretty quickly, so won't have any lingering effects on baby after birth. It also means that you need to keep it up for it to be effective. It is usually available on a wall outlet in most hospital labour wards, but can also come in portable canisters. There is generally a mixing valve, which means you can also turn it up or down to get what you need. It is something partners can help with by holding the tubing and passing the mouthpiece when needed for the next contraction.

Morphine shots – Morphine is a strong painkiller injected into the muscle or under the skin. Most Australian hospitals have moved to using morphine, but pethidine was the traditional drug of choice for labour in the past – and the occasional obstetrician will still keep it in the drug cupboard. The basic effect is the same. The morphine shot usually gives some relief for about 2–3 hours. Sometimes, a second shot can be given during labour, but if you are planning to only use a single morphine shot, you might want to save it for when you really need it. It tends to be good when your cervix is midway through opening (5–6 cm dilated), buying enough time to get you through to being ready to push. We don't like to give morphine shots when you are fully dilated (or close), because if the baby is born within an hour or so of a morphine shot, it can sometimes be a bit slower to breathe. This is easily reversible if it happens, but can be worrying for women to see their baby needing oxygen at birth. Given earlier in the labour, though, one or sometimes two shots of morphine will not have a significant impact on baby.

Patient controlled analgesia (PCA) – This option is not commonly used in Australian hospitals, but has a very important role for women who are unable to have an epidural and need strong pain relief for the duration of a labour. Known as 'the button', it is basically a way to give a small dose of a shorter-acting strong painkiller (such as remifentanil) through an intravenous drip. The button should only be pushed by the woman, and will lock out if it is pressed too many times in too short a period. This avoids being able to have too much of the drug. As the drug gets into the bloodstream, it can cross the placenta and have some effect on baby similar to morphine and pethidine, but clears a lot quicker, so can be used until closer to delivery.

Local anaesthetic – An injection of local anaesthetic makes the skin of the vagina and perineum numb. This is most useful if an assisted birth is needed, or when stitches are needed after the birth. Some women request to have local anaesthetic put into the skin of the perineum before the head starts to crown at the opening. The downsides of local anaesthetic are that it needs to be put in with a needle, which can hurt, and it can occasionally cause some bleeding from the needle puncture site. The numbness will usually last for an hour or two, which should be plenty of time to get a baby out and put in some stitches. Some obstetricians will be able to use local anaesthetic to block pain from the major nerve that covers the whole lower vagina and outer skin. This requires a long needle that is guided inside the vagina to the side of the pelvis. This is called a pudendal nerve block and, when done well, provides complete numbness to the vagina, which can be very useful for more complicated deliveries.

Epidural – The epidural is the ultimate pain reliever in labour. A needle is placed between the lower vertebrae just outside the spinal cord, with a tiny tube that delivers small amounts of anaesthetic to dull the nerves from that part of the spine down. To a lot of women, this sounds like a very scary prospect, but it is also very commonly used (around 1 in 3 births in Australia). With an effective epidural, you can get through labour feeling absolutely nothing. This can also be the problem, though. Not being able to feel pain usually means not being able to move either. If you have an epidural, you are going to need to stay on the bed for the rest of the labour. You will also have no control over your bladder, so a catheter will need to be put in to keep your bladder empty. Epidural anaesthetics don't directly pass into the blood or cross the placenta, so won't have a direct effect on baby. They can, however, have an effect on your blood pressure, which can have an effect on baby if the placenta does not get enough blood. For this reason, if you have an epidural, you will also need to have a monitor on for the baby's heartbeat.

Spinal anaesthetic – This is similar to an epidural, but uses a thinner needle, which is put slightly closer to the spine. A single dose of the anaesthetic is then injected. There is no tube coming out after, like an epidural, so repeat doses can't be given, but the effect is usually a lot stronger. It gives 1–2 hours of very good numbness. This is the most common anaesthetic used to perform caesarean section delivery, particularly if the caesarean is planned, and no epidural has been put in first.

Will acupuncture bring on labour?

Although there is no scientific evidence to suggest that acupuncture can bring on labour, it doesn't mean that it isn't a good idea for relaxation and wellness in preparation for birth. It may help you to relax and relieve any anxiety you may be experiencing leading up to the birth of your little one.

INDUCTION OF LABOUR

This is where you come into hospital and the doctor or midwife helps get you into labour. There are pros and cons to induction of labour, depending on the reason it is being offered. In general, the big plus is that the baby comes out earlier, and close to the day it is planned. This can be very important if the labour is expected to be very quick, if the woman lives at a distance from the hospital, or there are some possible risks at the start of labour that need to be watched for in a controlled environment.

There are some downsides. On average, induced labours are longer than natural labours (or, at least the intense part is). Women being induced are more likely to request medication to control pain, or an epidural. Whether it is actually more painful is a question that is subjective, and hard to answer. Because an induction is 'being done to you' rather than 'happening from within', it is natural to feel the response as pain. There is a chance that the medication being used to start the labour can put stress on the baby, so monitoring of the baby's heart has to be done more frequently, or sometimes continuously, in an induced labour.

It is a common misconception that induced labour makes it more likely that you will need a caesarean delivery (see page 214) or a forceps or vacuum birth (see page 209). In a lot of circumstances (including when a woman is overdue), research actually shows that timely induction of labour decreases the risk of caesarean birth and does not change the risk of forceps or vacuum birth at all.

Some of the reasons that an induction of labour may be offered are:

- You are more than a week overdue.
- Your baby has stopped growing.
- Your baby has a condition that requires it to be born with special staff in attendance, or in a specialised unit.
- You have diabetes.
- You have high blood pressure, or preeclampsia.
- There are good reasons related to home and family commitments.
- You have a pain condition, such as pubic symphysis separation.
- You are over 40 years of age and close to your due date.

So how is labour induced? During a normal labour, there are three things that have to happen: 1) Your uterus starts contracting; 2) Your cervix starts dilating; 3) Your waters break. In a natural labour, these three things can happen in any order, or all at the same time. Most commonly, it happens roughly in the order above. With an induced labour, these things need to happen in a specific order, and we have ways of helping each step along. It may be possible to skip one or two steps, depending on the situation, how close to the due date (or overdue) you are, or how many babies you have previously had.

STEP 1 – OPENING YOUR CERVIX

The first thing is for your cervix to be soft and open, ideally to at least 2 cm. If needed, this can be the longest step. When you are not pregnant, your cervix is a firm tube that is about 3–4 cm long, and only about half a centimetre wide. During the final weeks of pregnancy, as the baby's head presses down, the cervix becomes softer and starts to shorten in length. As it gets shorter, it starts to open from the inside, becoming more of a funnel shape. The direction of the cervix changes so that it is more in line with the vaginal opening, whereas it was previously facing back towards the tailbone (coccyx). The end of the cervix in the vagina starts to open last. This opening is called dilatation, which most people tend to focus on, but all the other changes are also important. We call all of the pre-labour changes to the cervix 'ripening'.

How ripe your cervix is can be quantified with a score system based on the things mentioned above. This is called a Bishop score. It is given as a number between 0 and 13 and takes into account not only how open your cervix is, but also how long it is, how soft it is, what direction it is facing and how low the baby's head is. Anything 6 or above is generally good to go for labour.

If your cervix is not ripe, you will need some help getting things started. The two methods of preparing the cervix for labour are to use hormonal medication called prostaglandins, or to mechanically stretch the cervix with a balloon. With either method, often you will be admitted to hospital the night before you plan to be in labour and your cervix will be ripened overnight. Sometimes, the cervix can be a bit stubborn. It is not uncommon for women to need to spend 2 or more nights in hospital waiting for the cervix to respond and open up.

Ripening the cervix with a hormone is the more commonly used method. This is because it is easier and usually more comfortable. The hormone either comes in a gel form or embedded in a plastic strip on the end of a string. Either way, it needs to be placed in the vagina, close to the top so it is alongside the cervix, where it needs to be working. The prostaglandin medication has a small chance of causing your uterus to contract strongly or too quickly, which is why most obstetricians will ask you to stay in hospital after it is given. There are a few things that might make prostaglandin induction riskier, including if the baby is very small, if the head of the baby is not low enough, or if you have previously had a caesarean delivery. A balloon induction can be useful in these circumstances.

With a balloon induction, the doctor usually uses a speculum to see your cervix. A thin rubber tube is threaded into the cervix, then a soft balloon on the end of the tube is inflated with sterile water until it is applying pressure on the cervix (up to 60–80 ml). Some devices have a second balloon that is filled up on the other side of the cervix inside the vagina. Either way, after the hormone or balloon is sited, you will be encouraged to get some rest. If you get cramps or have trouble sleeping, some painkillers or a mild sleeping tablet will generally be offered. It is important to get some sleep the first night of an induction, because the hard work usually starts the next day.

STEP 2 – BREAKING YOUR WATERS

When your cervix is soft, open and ready for labour, the next step is 'letting the plug out of the baby bath'. In a labour that has started naturally, a lot of women like to delay breaking the waters as long as possible. Most of the time, it is just an inevitable part of natural labour anyway. There are pros and cons to deliberately letting the amniotic fluid out. When the waters break, whether the labour is natural-onset or being induced, it will almost always cause the uterus to contract more strongly. There are a few reasons for this.

The release of fluid causes the uterus to shrink in around the baby. This gives the muscle of the uterus more ability to squeeze, a bit like a water balloon. If it is overfull, squeezing at the top will not change the shape of the balloon as much as it would if you let half the water out. The fluid comes out from the cervix and, naturally, whatever is above the cervix (usually the baby's head) will come down more strongly on it to 'plug the hole'. This increased stretch on the cervix also increases contractions by a nerve reflex. So the head pushes on the cervix, which stretches it. The stretch on the cervix tells the uterus to squeeze harder. The harder the uterus squeezes, the more firmly the head pushes on the cervix. And so on . . .

After the waters break, often labour will already start to happen on its own. Everybody and every baby is different, though. For a woman who has had a few babies before, and where there is a huge gush of fluid released, this might only take a few minutes to work. If it is the woman's first baby and only a trickle of fluid comes out, the natural effect might take a day or two. Most of the time, when we start an induction, we like to keep things moving, so after breaking the waters it will usually be suggested to start the next step of the induction to get active labour started.

The actual breaking of the waters is called an ARM, for artificial rupture of the membranes. The doctor or midwife will need to do an internal check to feel your cervix and make sure it is open. They then pass a long, plastic stick, with a tiny sharp hook on the end, along their fingers until it gets to the opening in the cervix. More colloquially, this is often called 'the crochet hook'. It looks scarier than it is. The tiny hook on the end would be barely able to break the skin if you tried to scratch yourself with it. The reason it is so long is to give a bit of leverage, but the tip only needs to go about 5–6 cm into the vagina. Most of the time, it takes less than 30 seconds to break the waters, and there are no nerves in the amniotic sac, so it shouldn't hurt much more than a normal internal check.

In reality, sometimes it can be a little bit trickier to break the waters. If you have a less experienced doctor or midwife, they may need to have a couple of tries, or call somebody else to have another go. There can be a small amount of blood after this procedure as well, because the cervix has fragile glands lining it that can easily spot blood when stretched.

The amount of amniotic fluid is variable. It may be half a cup, or it may be over a litre. The midwife or doctor will usually comment on the colour of the fluid (clear or pink is good) and you will be asked to have the monitor put on to listen to the baby's heart for a while after the waters have broken.

STEP 3 – MAKING YOUR UTERUS CONTRACT

Sometimes, one or both of the above steps will be all that is needed, and labour will start of its own accord. Other times, the steps happen naturally, but no contractions follow and we need to help make them come. There is only one treatment we use to start contractions: oxytocin. Oxytocin is a hormone that is naturally produced from a part of your brain called the pituitary gland. It is always elevated in the blood during natural labour. When it flows into the blood of your uterus, it causes it to contract. It is a short-acting hormone, so needs to be continuously released into the blood to keep being effective.

The oxytocin used to artificially induce contractions is chemically identical to that produced by your brain. It is given through an intravenous line, and made very dilute with saline. The amount your body might need to get the uterus contracting is variable, so oxytocin is started slowly, and increased gradually until the contractions are strong and frequent enough. Most hospitals have set instructions for midwives about how quickly to increase the oxytocin when it is used for induction, to avoid contractions getting too intense too suddenly.

When oxytocin is given artificially, the uterus can contract quicker and stronger than it would otherwise in a natural labour. When we use it, we need to be careful to avoid this. This risk also means we need to continuously listen to the baby's heartbeat. If the amount of oxytocin is more than you need, you will usually know, as the contractions will be too intense. If you have an epidural, you may not be able to feel the contractions and can't tell the doctor or midwife if it is too intense. Having a monitor (CTG) on while an oxytocin infusion is happening also allows us to see how often each contraction is coming and how long it is lasting. By looking at this and the pattern of the baby's heartbeat we are able to make sure oxytocin is used safely.

The need to be 'strapped down' on a monitor, with an IV line, is a major downside of induced labour. With modern, wireless CTG monitors and motivated support people, it is possible to stay mobile, use the shower and even a birthing pool while making safe, monitored use of oxytocin. Some women are fearful of oxytocin use in hospitals. But it is not the oxytocin itself that is dangerous. When naturally made from your brain, it is celebrated – some people call it the 'love drug'. When oxytocin is used to induce or speed up labour, it needs to be used respectfully. There are some vocal people who like to refer to a 'cascade of intervention', of which oxytocin is the catalyst. On the flipside, oxytocin use saves lives on a daily basis around the world, both in labour and after birth, and is listed on the World Health Organization's list of essential medicines for safety in healthcare.

STEP 4 – LABOUR AS YOU HAD PLANNED (MORE OR LESS)

After that, you are free to labour as you had planned. As mentioned in step three, if you end up with the oxytocin drip, there is the extra requirement of monitoring and the IV line, which can be an inconvenience. Keep in mind that these things may well be recommended even in a labour that has started of its own accord.

Augmentation of labour

Oxytocin is often used to speed up a labour that has started naturally but slowed or stopped for various reasons. In this circumstance we call it augmentation rather than induction. Essentially, an augmented labour is step two or three used during a labour that started on its own. Augmenting labour, by breaking the waters or using an oxytocin drip, is often feared by patients. In general, augmenting labour will make the total duration of labour much quicker (in contrast to induction, which can be on average a bit longer). Augmentation will make things more intense and increase the likelihood of using pain-relief medication. Augmentation of labour (when done for the right reasons) is generally accepted to increase the chances of vaginal delivery.

The concept of augmenting labour as 'interfering' with a natural process does have merit in some respects. Certainly, induction or augmentation needs to be respected as a medical intervention and should only be done when necessary and with the woman's understanding and acceptance of the reasons. Medical intervention to start or speed up labour is not, in itself, the reason that Australian babies are now more likely to be born by caesarean than they were 30 years ago. Compared with developing countries, there is no doubt that access to these medical interventions is the reason that Australian rates of major complications for mothers and babies are amongst the lowest in the world. In general, it shouldn't be anything to be feared, but you should also be satisfied that it is being offered for the right reasons.

LABOUR AND BIRTH

Traditionally, labour is divided into three stages. In simple terms these are:

- First stage – the time when you start getting contractions, up until when you are ready to push.
- Second stage – when you are ready to push the baby out (when the cervix is fully dilated), up until the baby actually does come out.
- Third stage – after the baby is out until it is all over. This is basically getting the placenta out and making sure your uterus contracts.

Keep in mind that things can vary greatly between women and labours. The experience of a first labour is also, on average, a lot longer than that of somebody who has already had a few babies. In fact, one medical book I read in my training started by saying: 'Primipara and Multipara should be regarded as two different species.'

FIRST STAGE

Labour can start very slowly or be very sudden. Usually, if you have to ask 'Am I in labour?', the answer is most likely: 'Not quite yet.'

A very common question for women preparing for their first birth is: 'How will I know when I am in labour?' There is an ancient medical definition of labour – *'the presence of painful uterine contractions associated with change in the cervix over time'*. So having the uterus contract (go rock hard), is definitely a part of it. Pain is subjective, but there should definitely be another level above the Braxton Hicks practice contractions, which are usually happening in the lead-up. When I am asked how often contractions should be coming and how long they should be lasting for, a reasonable benchmark for early labour is regular contractions less than 5 minutes apart and for more than 30 seconds when they come. In the intense part of labour, these should be closer to 3 minutes apart and lasting up to a minute.

I have found the most reliable and quick indication that a woman is in labour is her ignoring everyone and everything around her during a contraction. This doesn't have to be screaming, crying or swearing (all of which are common coping mechanisms in labour). Many women simply close their eyes, look away or tense their face a little bit. Without fail though, any woman in true labour (without an epidural) will stop whatever they were doing or saying – mid-sentence – the moment a true labour contraction starts.

To know how effective these contractions are at causing your cervix to dilate, a vaginal examination is needed. How frequently examinations are done is something every woman should talk to their doctor or midwife about. Some practitioners are happy to manage labour without examinations, waiting to follow a woman's own instincts. The progress of labour can also be determined by watching changes in her behaviour, or by feeling the abdomen and checking how low the head has dropped from the top, but there would be very few midwives or obstetricians who would say they *never* do vaginal examinations in labour.

The typical frequency of vaginal examinations in labour is every 4 hours, or at any time if there are signs that things have changed (like a desire to push, a change in the baby's heart rhythm or the fluid coming out). How dilated you are, as well as other information about the progress of labour, is recorded on a graph called a partogram. The idea of putting progress of labour down into a set formula of dilation versus time is a little bit overly simplified and old-fashioned, but it does give a good indication of how labour has been going and is a useful tool when multiple care providers need to be involved over the course of your labour.

Labour is basically an arduous count to 10. Most women get very focused on the number you give them after an examination, because each centimetre is one step closer to that magical 10, or fully dilated.

Vaginal examination in labour

When a doctor or midwife does a vaginal examination in labour, they are placing two sterile gloved fingers into the vagina and feeling as deep as they need to in order to reach your cervix. By moving the fingers apart inside the cervix, they are able to estimate how dilated the cervix is. Beyond the cervix, they will be able to feel the top of baby's head, or the bag of waters if these have not yet broken.

During a vaginal examination, the doctor or midwife will check the following:

The cervix: dilatation

For most women, the big question is: 'How dilated am I?' How open the cervix has become during labour is a good indication that you are making progress. It is one of the many factors that are assessed during a vaginal examination. Apart from opening up, the cervix also has to shorten down, called 'effacement'. A very short, thin cervix is a much better sign than a long thick cervix, even if it is not as open. How soft and stretchy the cervix is can also be felt, which gives a good idea of how easily the cervix will continue to open up. Sometimes, if a woman is stuck in mid-labour, the cervix may become swollen (oedematous), which can indicate that the baby is coming down in a position that is putting uneven pressure on the cervix.

The descent: station

How low the baby has come down in the birth canal is felt by placing one finger on the baby's head and using the other finger to feel for a pointy bone on the side of the pelvis (called 'ischial spines'). We talk about 'station' of the baby's head, which is how close the baby is to this pointy part, either behind or in front. If the top of baby's head is past the pointy part (referred to as +1 or +2), this is a good sign that the baby is coming down well and shouldn't be too tight a fit. The pointy parts are at the narrowest part of the pelvis. Once the mid-point of baby's head is past them, the hardest part is over. This generally does not happen until the pushing stage. In many ways, how low the baby's head is can be more significant than how dilated the cervix is.

Position of the baby's head

The part of the examination that takes the longest is feeling the baby's scalp. (This should still all be less than 30 seconds – though I'm sure that feels like 30 seconds too many when you are in labour.) There is a lot of information that can be gained from the feel of a baby's head in labour. The skull is made up of many bones that are, more or less, fused together by the time you are an adult. The bones in the skull of a baby are not joined yet and are able to squeeze together and overlap. This is nature's small mercy for women in labour, as it allows the total size of baby's head to be that little bit smaller to push out.

During a vaginal examination in labour, we are able to feel the gaps between the bones on the baby's skull. The line between bones are called sutures, and the soft spots where the bones meet are called fontanelles. At the top of baby's forehead, four bones meet. At this point, there are four lines (sutures) coming together, and the soft spot (anterior fontanelle) is shaped like a diamond. At the back of baby's head, there are three lines coming together, and the soft spot (posterior fontanelle) is not really soft at all, but feels like the top of a triangle, or an arrow shape.

The easiest way for baby to get out is if it is facing your tailbone, with its chin tucked down so that the back of its head is coming under the pubic bone. This is called flexed occipito-anterior position. This is when we feel the arrow-shaped part of the head directly in the middle, and the arrow is pointing down. The harder way for baby to get out is if it is looking up toward the pubic region and has its neck stretched out. We call this deflexed occipito-posterior position. By feel, this is more likely if we can easily feel the diamond-shaped spot on the baby's head and the line down the middle of the forehead.

In short: triangle good; diamond bad.

We are also feeling for that overlap of the baby's skull bones. How close the bones are indicates how much pressure the baby is getting from the contractions, and how tight the fit is in your pelvis. This is called moulding of the head. There is also a natural swelling on top of the baby's head, where fluid gets trapped under the skin from the pressure, called 'caput'. The combination of these things can help us tell if baby is a bit wedged in, or if your contractions are strong enough.

When your baby is born, the shape of the head will often be a bit elongated and the top of the head will feel a bit squishy. This is normal. It will return to a nice rounded shape in a couple of days.

How quickly will I dilate?

When the intense part of labour has begun, the average rate of dilatation is around 1 cm per hour. This can be much quicker, and usually is much quicker when it is not your first baby. It can also be slower, and 1 cm every 2 hours is generally thought to be an acceptable speed of natural dilatation. The idea that the cervix dilates at a set rate is fairly artificial. In reality, the cervix dilates at a more random pace with periods of quicker and slower dilatation throughout the course of labour. In general, it is a good thing if the cervix is a bit more open with every check, and the baby's head is a bit lower.

What will happen if I stop dilating?

If things seem to have stopped or slowed down, the doctor or midwife may suggest some ways of getting labour back on track. The methods used are similar to those used to induce labour (see page 176). Sometimes, something as simple as a change in your position can be very helpful. Think of it as trying to thread a nut onto a bolt – if things seem a bit tight, often jiggling things a little bit helps to find the right angle for things to keep going. In more difficult labours, the analogy of fitting a square peg into a round hole might be better. By changing posture, such as moving from lying to standing, or turning to all fours or a kneeling position, you are altering the effect of gravity on the baby in your womb. Also, by changing the angle of your pelvis in relation to your spine, you are able to give the baby better options to get its head into the best position to fit through your pelvis.

If labour contractions have slowed as dilatation slows down, a couple of interventions will often be recommended to bring contractions back. This is often referred to as augmentation of labour (see page 181). The simplest way to increase the strength and frequency of contractions is to break the waters. Releasing the amniotic fluid reduces the space around the baby in the womb. This allows the muscle of the uterus to squeeze harder. It also increases the force of the baby's head down onto the cervix, which improves dilatation. The arguments against breaking the waters are that it can sometimes reinforce a bad position of the baby, as it will have less room to move into an optimal position for birth. The other possibility after the waters break is that the umbilical cord may be in a position where more pressure is applied to it with contractions, which can cause changes in the baby's heart rate that will need to be watched.

The waters breaking is a natural part of labour, though, and will have to happen at some point (even if it is immediately before the birth). If your doctor or midwife is suggesting that your waters should be broken, they will have a discussion about the pros and cons. Be aware that after the waters break, it is natural for labour to become more intense, so you will need to be prepared for this.

The second way that labour contractions can be increased is by using an oxytocin infusion (see page 180). Use of oxytocin when labour has already begun should be done with care. If you are already in labour, it is important that the doctor or midwife has excluded any problems with the way that baby is coming down before making your contractions stronger. Compared with an oxytocin infusion to induce labour, its use during an already established labour has a potentially higher possibility of causing contractions to be too strong for your body or baby (called hyperstimulation). In particular, care should be taken if it is not your first baby, or if you have previously had a baby by caesarean section.

Occasionally, if contractions are good but things seem a bit jammed up, an epidural may be suggested to improve the progress of labour. This is definitely a double-edged sword, as it can cause the contractions to slow, requiring oxytocin to bring them back. In some situations, though, it allows the muscles in the pelvis to relax a bit more, which lets the baby come down further. It can also be useful if a woman has an overwhelming urge to push (called involuntary pushing) but the cervix is not fully dilated yet. In this situation, sometimes pushing can make the situation worse, and the numbing effect of the epidural takes away this urge.

How do I know my waters have broken?

You might think you have wet your pants, or maybe you wake in the middle of the night with water beneath you. The feeling of your waters breaking may be a slow warm trickle, or possibly a gush of fluid. The fluid is usually odourless and colourless. Some women say it has a distinct sweet, inoffensive smell. Unlike what you see in the movies, your waters breaking may not be the first sign of labour.

After your waters have broken, you will contact your midwife or the hospital, if you haven't already, and they may ask you a series of questions to gauge how far along you are in labour.

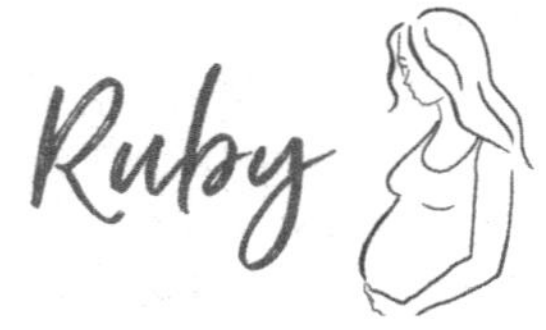

COPING WITH CONTRACTIONS

If your waters have broken but contractions haven't yet started or have begun to slow, you might be advised to stay at home, relax and rest until your labour progresses. The contractions typically start off in waves, and are similar to strong period pain.

A contraction lasts anywhere between 30 and 60 seconds. Contractions become progressively stronger over time, and the pain intensifies. This is when breathing techniques, movement, or taking a shower or a bath come into play. Once you are in the active phase of labour, contractions also become more frequent.

The transition phase may cause you to vomit, shake or tremble, feel withdrawn or become distressed. You may also start to feel hot or cold. The pressure down below becomes stronger as the baby's head moves down the birth canal.

Some things that may help you through the contractions are:

- Walking around, moving or rocking on an exercise ball. (If you have an epidural you won't be able to do this, but you're unlikely to feel the contractions anyway.)
- Water. A warm bath or shower can work as a relaxant and help to ease pain.
- Using relaxation techniques, such as breathing exercises.
- Getting your partner to massage your lower back.
- Using acupressure or a TENS machine (see page 171).

Timing contractions

You will need to time from when the contraction begins and how long the contraction lasts for. This is a good job to delegate to your support person.

There are many apps that you can download or you can simply write it down. When you call the maternity ward, they will most likely ask you how far apart your contractions are and how long they go for.

When timing your contractions, start when a contraction begins and stop at the beginning of the next contraction.

Things a partner or support person can do to help during birth:

- Being empathic and doing your best to understand what she is experiencing is the most important thing you can do to help her through both the pregnancy and birth.
- Don't stress if you don't get around to reading parenting books, but do join your partner in the antenatal classes if you can. This is an excellent way to prepare you for what will happen at the birth.
- Draw up the birth plan together. If your partner is unable to advocate for herself at any point during labour, you can make decisions in line with her wishes and ensure her choices are respected.
- Providing your partner with reassurance and positivity – even just holding her hand and telling her she's doing brilliantly – can be a great deal of support throughout labour.
- Seeing your partner in so much pain can be confronting. Sometimes, stepping outside for a moment to take a breather and calm yourself can help.

David

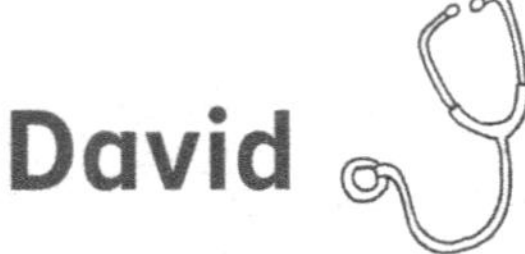

How do we know that baby is coping with labour?

This is one of the most important roles of a midwife or obstetrician. Making sure baby is okay is our thing, so you don't need to be focused on that. All you need to focus on is coping with labour yourself.

Labour is a stressful time, not just for the woman but also for the baby. During labour and birth, the baby has suddenly had all its warm fluid drained. It is then repetitively squeezed and its head pushed down and adjusted to the fit of the mother's pelvis. Meanwhile, its lifeline (the umbilical cord) may be compressed, wrapped and tangled. The placenta is also being put to the test.

Baby's placenta is its makeshift all-in-one organ – lungs, gut and kidneys. It is nature's life-support system. Up until labour begins, this amazing organ is constantly bathed in a stream of mother's blood, allowing passage of oxygen and nutrients in, and toxins and waste material out.

During the contractions of labour, the giant muscle of the uterus squeezes for up to 60 seconds at a time. During this time, blood flow to the placenta is restricted. Once the contraction ends, new blood rushes in under the placenta to replace the blood that was trapped there during the contraction. Think of it like holding your breath. During the contraction, the baby is essentially holding its breath. After the contraction, it uses the time before the next one to catch its breath. In this way, from the baby's point of view, labour can be compared to a marathon. Whether it is a short or a long marathon depends on the woman. How fit the placenta is to run this marathon is partly a question of the mother's health, but there are also a lot of factors completely out of anybody's control.

The big fear with monitoring a baby during labour comes down to one thing: is baby getting enough oxygen to its brain? There are a few features of labour that can give us some indication of how the baby is doing, such as the baby's movements, the colour of the fluid and whether the mother has normal vital signs and temperature. These things can give us an idea of how baby is doing, and whether or not there is any reason to suspect a baby might not be coping.

When we need to answer that big question, though, there are only two tests we use: cardiotocography (CTG) and fetal scalp blood sampling.

Cardiotocography (CTG) – continuous fetal heart rate monitoring

Most women experience this during their pregnancy or labour, for one reason or another. It is sometimes referred to as 'the straps' (by patients) or 'the monitor' (by staff). Most machines in Australia are similar, consisting of two circular discs like teacup saucers, which are held in place over the tummy with elastic straps. One of these discs hears the heartbeat, while the other one picks up changes in pressure, and can tell us when a contraction is happening. The information from these sensors is printed out on a strip of paper continuously (or to a computer program and screen). This allows a doctor or midwife to observe changes in the heart pattern of the baby over time, and in relation to any contractions. This reading is sometimes referred to as 'the trace'. More modern machines are wireless, meaning that the sensors can be strapped to the tummy, but do not have to be directly connected to the machine. A lot are also waterproof, meaning that the woman can still enter the shower or a birthing pool if she wants to, even if continuous heart monitoring has been recommended.

CTG has a single major advantage over listening to the baby intermittently, as a midwife or doctor is likely to know if the baby is under significant stress. In theory, this reduces the chances of a baby suffering labour-related brain damage from lack of oxygen (one of the possible causes of cerebral palsy). There are certainly cases where unwell babies, despite continuous monitoring, go unrecognised, but most of these cases are a result of human error. In general, this is a very sensitive test for a baby who is not coping with labour due to lack of oxygen.

There are numerous disadvantages, however. It is uncomfortable for a labouring woman to have straps on her abdomen, and the sound of the baby's heart, though often reassuring and soothing, can also be a cause of stress. The most significant problem with CTG is that changes in the heart pattern are often caused by other stresses in labour that are not a long-term concern for baby. For this reason, doctors or midwives may act on a suspicious CTG pattern and call for urgent delivery, only to find that the baby was fine all along. This is why a CTG often goes hand-in-hand with the reputation for staff in hospitals over-intervening with caesarean or other procedures.

The term for this is 'specificity'. A CTG is sensitive to detecting a baby under stress. It is not necessarily specific as to what that stress is from. There are some ways to limit intervention from CTG, such as only using the device when there is a risk factor for baby, and increasing staff education in interpreting patterns. It is recognised that use of CTG increases caesarean rates. It is also accepted that it decreases the incidence of brain damage due to unrecognised lack of oxygen. There is a grey zone, where potentially some unnecessary caesareans can be avoided, but reassurance that baby is still coping is still required. This is where fetal scalp blood sampling has a role.

Fetal scalp blood sampling

The idea of this is worse than the reality. If it is suspected that a baby is not coping with labour, but we cannot be certain based on the heart rate pattern alone, another method is used to reassure that emergency delivery is not required. A tiny blood sample from baby can give us information about how the baby is metabolising and whether it is likely to be struggling with getting enough oxygen. When our bodies are working hard without enough oxygen, a by-product of metabolism is lactic acid. Another effect of this is that blood acidity changes. If these levels are changing, it is much more likely the baby is under significant stress needing immediate delivery. If these blood measures are normal, we can be reassured it is safe to continue with labour.

To take a blood sample, the most accessible part of the baby is usually the top of baby's head. We use a device a bit like a circular speculum, put a bit of Vaseline on baby's head, then make a pin-prick. The little drop of blood is sucked up in a thin tube, which is then analysed for pH and lactate. For an experienced doctor, this should only take a few minutes. Having this done is a little bit intense, but in the right situation, it can save an unnecessary caesarean. For a woman in labour who may be presented with an ultimatum for a caesarean birth due to fetal distress, it can be worth knowing about this test and asking if it is appropriate for her situation. It is generally quite safe and does not leave marks on the baby. The main reasons the test would not be used include knowledge of a blood-borne virus carried by the mother, such as hepatitis, or a known problem with blood clotting that could possibly be affecting the baby, such as haemophilia, or extremely low platelets.

SECOND STAGE

This is the business end of labour. This is the part in all the movies, where the woman screams and the partner passes out, and it's all over in a few minutes . . . It's not usually like the movies at all.

From the time you are ready to push until the time the baby comes out is usually a couple of hours in first labours. It is also completely normal to need to actively push for over an hour, even up to 2 hours, before baby comes out. This part does get quicker the more babies you have. It is not uncommon for this part to only be two or three pushes in somebody who has had a few babies.

When you are almost ready to push, baby's head starts to fully come through the cervix and tends to drop deeper into the birth canal. This part of labour is called transition. It tends to be the most intense part (second, maybe, to crowning, or just before the head comes out). The good news is once you are fully dilated, the intensity usually decreases again. Once you are fully dilated, you will often notice a new pressure on the pelvic floor. Most women describe this feeling like needing to poo. This is because the baby's head is pressing on your rectum. This pressure is probably the baby. It could also be both.

Am I going to poo?

The odds are pretty high that you will; it's totally natural. You are just going to have to let it happen. Obstetricians and midwives expect it, so don't worry. It is also something that will be dealt with very discreetly. The birth attendant will usually wipe it away before anybody has much of a chance to notice it. You can't hold in a poo and push out a baby out at the same time: it is a physical impossibility. Relaxing about the whole thing will help a lot because (to quote every midwife ever) when you push a baby out, you have to *push down like you are doing a big poo.* This is almost a universal thing that midwives say in the second stage (except in the movies!).

I often tell women to 'push with your diaphragm' and 'let everything down there relax'. The modern trend is to tell women to 'follow your natural instincts'. That is totally fine if baby is coming whether you like it or not, but some people aren't that lucky.

How to push

These days nobody really tells pregnant women 'how' to push during check-ups or antenatal classes, but they do during labour. So, having observed many, many deliveries, but never having done it myself, I will attempt to summarise how to push out a baby:

- **Use your diaphragm and abdominal muscles.** It is hard to apply strong force down to your pelvic floor while breathing in and out. To effectively use your diaphragm (the muscle under your lungs), you kind of need to hold your breath. Some clinicians teach women breathing techniques that allow them to push while taking long breaths. In general though, it is advisable to push until you are red in the face.
- **Let the muscles of your thighs, bottom and hips relax.** Sometimes, it can be useful to bring the knees up higher than the hips. This can be achieved in an upright position by squatting, and is also the principle behind the birth stool.
- **Arch your lower back.** This opens the angle between your lower spine and your pelvis. This can be achieved on all fours, or in kneeling or squatting birthing positions. When lying on a bed, it can also be achieved in stirrups. Lying down with legs in the air actually puts your spine and pelvis into a similar position as squatting, just rotated from vertical to horizontal, and losing the assistance of gravity. The reason it gets a bad rap is because obstetricians usually get women into this position when they are about to use intervention, like forceps.
- **Keep up the momentum.** We often say something like, 'quick breath, then go again'. When you are pushing well, the idea is to keep it up. Rather than have a good push, then relax and let the baby slip back, try to stack the pushes close together during the contraction. Some practitioners will ask you to do 'three good pushes' during your contraction. In your head, count to 10 during each push to make them nice and long. Also, remember your last push during a contraction is usually your best – so make it count.
- **Be patient.** It takes time. Especially the first baby. I will often tell women when they start pushing that their job is to move the baby a total of 2 or 3 cm. Every time they push during a contraction, they may move it 3 mm forward, then it will slip 2 mm backwards, so it

could take 30 contractions before the baby is out. It is tempting to ask the doctor to 'pull it out'. A good birth clinician should always be assessing to see that you are making steady progress. Listen to the doctor or midwife: if they say you are making progress, they are (probably) telling you the truth. Sometimes using a mirror or feeling the top of baby's head will help give you the motivation that your pushes really *are* doing something.

- When they say 'Stop pushing!' . . . STOP PUSHING. This is because the last part of getting baby out tends to happen pretty quickly. All the effort is mainly to get the widest part of the baby's skull through the narrowest part of the bones of your pelvis. After this point, all that remains is the soft, swollen tissue of your pelvic floor. Midwives debate about a 'hands on' or 'hands off' approach to getting the baby safely over your perineum. It is, however, pretty widely accepted that, when it comes to crowning, slower is better. If the person delivering your baby wants you to stop pushing, it is because they want to slow down the baby's progress over your perineum to try to prevent a tear. It is obviously easier to say than do though. Common techniques to deal with this part including panting, or long breaths. The idea is to give your pelvic floor enough time to get over the initial shock of the stretch, and to relax rather than tense up as the baby comes through.
- If you say 'I can't do this!', odds are you are just about to do it. It may just be my observation, but the moment women reach this point of frustration or despair is often the same moment something just *clicks*. Maybe it is a second wind, or maybe it is because the head just got that bit lower and suddenly it is dawning how the baby comes out. Either way, if you hear yourself saying something like this, it's probably about to happen.
- There is no right way to push. After saying all of the above, I am just going to throw it right out again. The truth is, I have seen babies come out with all sorts of things going on with the mother. Some swear or scream it out. Vomiting is surprisingly good. A lot of babies come out on the toilet when the mother thought they had to push for something else. Some women even manage to barely say or do anything, almost with a Mona Lisa smile. In a lot of cases, baby is going to come out no matter what you do. The tips above are mainly for if it doesn't happen, without overthinking it.

After the baby's head is out, the rest of the baby should emerge with the next contraction. During this time, the baby often will naturally turn its head back to the side, so it is in a more natural alignment with the spine, called restitution. If the baby does not come out with a push during the next contraction, the clinician will place a hand on each side of the baby's head and direct force downwards until they can see the tip of baby's shoulder coming out. Then they will change direction and apply force upwards to get the other shoulder out. If this doesn't happen fairly quickly, it can lead to shoulder dystocia (see page 208).

After the shoulders, the baby comes out super quickly. In the very first moments of life, baby may look a little blue and may not immediately start to cry or breathe. This is often normal, and the doctor or midwife present will be keeping an eye out to make sure that baby springs into life within a normal timeframe. Usually, baby will be brought directly up onto your stomach or chest, to give baby 'skin-to-skin', which is where the baby can directly feel your touch. There are plenty of benefits to this, which are beyond the scope of this section. Just know skin-to-skin is good. So be prepared to get messy.

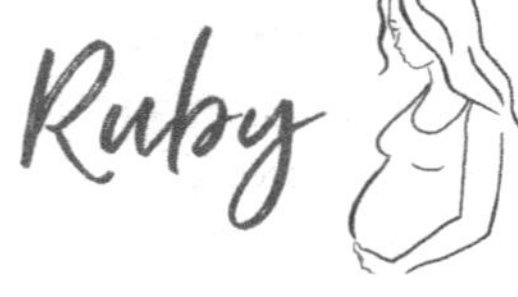

How it feels to push

Once you are 10 cm dilated, your doctor or midwife will encourage you to try and push. If you have an epidural, you may need some direction as to when to push. When I interviewed friends and family members about how they would describe pushing or bearing down (with no epidural), most described feeling that their body instinctively knew what to do – almost as though they couldn't stop themselves. Many spoke of the need to moan or grunt as they pushed. Some said they experienced a sensation of burning as the baby's head was crowning.

Everyone said: in this moment, nothing else matters. You forget about the fact that midwives and doctors are looking at your lady parts; you certainly forget about how you look! You may feel overcome with emotion by the intensity of the moment, and then feel a profound relief when your baby takes its first breath.

What I'm really thinking:

Giving birth

Throughout the writing of this book, I spoke to countless women about their pregnancies but mostly their birth stories. Maybe it is what connects mothers to each other. Possibly, it could be for validation or the need to embrace what happened during those defining moments, or maybe it is because it still generally isn't a topic that is freely spoken about. I chatted with women from all backgrounds: women who gave birth in birthing centres, at home, in the bath; others who had elective or emergency C-sections. Some delivered babies that were born posterior, others breech.

Many women spoke of a beautiful, empowering birth and said they could do it over and over again; many others told me how the birth didn't go to plan; some revealed traumatic experiences and how afterwards they needed time to heal, both physically and emotionally.

Giving birth – bringing new life into the world, no matter how you do it – is such an incredible moment for you and your partner. We should never feel as though we have 'failed'. We all handle the birthing experience differently. No two births are the same.

There is no right or wrong way to give birth and your experience will be just that: *your* experience. That's the thing about birth, it is purely our own experience, soon to be a memory but never to be forgotten.

David

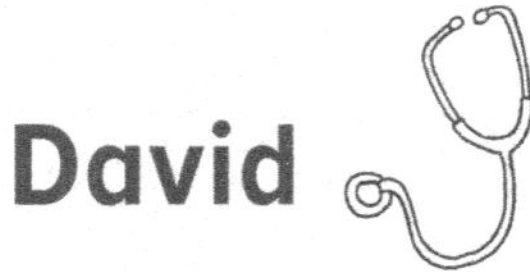

THIRD STAGE

Baby is out in the world! Hopefully, he or she has had a nice loud cry and is starting to turn pink. There is still the matter of that cord going down between your legs, and the placenta still inside your womb.

Cutting the cord

At some point, it will generally be suggested to cut the cord. Some families prefer to not cut the cord at all, but let the cord and placenta fall off naturally in time. This is called a lotus birth. Delayed cord clamping is more commonly requested, where we wait until it has completely stopped pulsating before cutting.

There is some evidence that waiting for the cord to stop before cutting it can be beneficial for the baby, particularly if it is a bit premature. Until the cord stops pulsating, blood from the baby is still being passed through the placenta. If the baby is crying or breathing quietly, there is no need for blood to be going through the placenta for the sake of getting oxygen to the baby. As the physiology of the baby catches up and realises this is no longer necessary, the vessels in the cord spasm and blood stops moving through the placenta. This happens relatively quickly, and most umbilical cords have stopped pulsating within about 5 minutes of the birth.

Babies in the womb have a higher total blood volume than they need to survive outside the womb. This is because at any given time, a significant volume of this blood will be in the placental vessels. It is normal for some of this blood to stay in the placenta after birth. By delaying clamping, the baby gets a bit more blood than they would if the cord were immediately cut. This can be a good thing if the baby needs more blood, such as with a degree of prematurity. It may also decrease a baby's risk of iron deficiency in its first few months.

A few conditions can be made a little bit worse if the baby has too much blood in its system. In this circumstance, delaying cord clamping may contribute to the need for treatment of a transient condition called neonatal jaundice. After birth, the haemoglobin in the baby's blood cells changes so that it is better at carrying blood from the lungs rather than the placenta. As part of this, some blood cells are naturally destroyed by the baby. When this happens, bilirubin is released into the bloodstream, which can make the skin or eyes turn a yellow colour. It can also make the baby drowsy and unwell. This is neonatal jaundice. It tends to happen 3 to 4 days after birth and then improves, but may need some additional observation and treatment, such as phototherapy, if it happens.

Another reason for not delaying the cord cutting is when the baby needs immediate help with breathing. It is much easier for the team attending your birth to help the baby (if needed) after it is separated from the placenta.

In practice, if the baby comes out healthy, I recommend couples cut the cord when it feels right. There is no rush, and no wrong time to do it. I usually wait until the couple have had plenty of time to enjoy those first moments.

Umbilical cord blood banking

Instead of the umbilical cord being discarded after birth, remaining blood can be collected from it and stored for use in the future. This blood is rich in stem cells and can be used in treating conditions in both children and adults that involve the immune system. Diseases that are most commonly treated using stem cells include leukaemia, blood diseases, metabolic diseases and immune deficiencies.

You can choose to donate the blood to the public cord blood bank, who use it for bone marrow treatments, or you can privately organise to store the blood for potential later uses. If you choose to bank your baby's blood, you will need to organise and pay for it prior to giving birth. It is important that you also discuss your intentions with your midwives and doctor.

Birthing the placenta

Once the cord is cut, the next step is getting the placenta out of the womb. This is also reasonably quick, and usually happens within the first 15 minutes after the birth. It can take up to an hour after the birth for the placenta to come away, but any longer than this is considered abnormal and may have potential dangers, particularly for bleeding.

In general, there are two ways that your midwife or doctor may suggest dealing with the placenta. The first is called physiological third stage, and is waiting for the placenta to come away naturally without any specific hands-on assistance from the clinician. Sometimes, the woman may have to do some pushing to get the placenta out of the vagina, but mostly this method is just a matter of being patient. The benefit of this approach is that it feels very natural and, in most situations, it will happen of its own accord, as the body is designed for this. Having baby directly on your skin, or attaching baby to the breast, can help your body to complete this process. One downside is that, by waiting for physiological third stage, the duration of the process may take a little longer. The other concern is that heavier bleeding can occur.

It is natural for bleeding to occur under the placenta during third stage, as this helps the placenta to separate and come away. Sometimes, if the placenta doesn't completely separate, bleeding can start and then continue until the placenta is out. This may be obvious, as a growing pool of blood between the woman's legs. It can sometimes not be obvious, if the blood gets trapped inside the womb or inside the amniotic sac from the baby. A midwife or doctor should still be able to recognise this by feeling for the level of your fundus (top of the womb), which should be somewhere around your belly button, and should not get much higher.

Due to this risk of bleeding, another method of helping the placenta come away is commonly recommended. This is referred to as active management of third stage. With active management, an injection of oxytocin is given to you shortly after the baby is born, usually in the thigh. This causes the afterbirth contractions to happen a bit sooner and makes them a bit stronger. Once the cord is cut and there are some signs that the placenta is starting to separate, such as a small gush of blood, or a change in the shape of the womb, the midwife or doctor will place one hand on your abdomen to support the womb.

Their other hand will apply gentle, continuous traction down on the umbilical cord. This is referred to as controlled cord traction.

The major benefit of active management is thought to be a reduction in the average amount of blood loss occurring after birth. For this reason, it is commonly the default management recommended by most public health systems in Australia. The main downsides perceived by patients are that it feels less natural, a medication is required to be given, and it may be a bit more uncomfortable. In practice, the medication given is oxytocin, the same hormone that your body is making to help push the placenta out naturally. A skilled clinician will give this injection quickly and subtly so that the woman barely notices it. The duration of contractions needed to help get the placenta out is usually only for 2 or 3 minutes and, if done well, this does not cause much discomfort. The overall time taken to get the placenta out is also much quicker.

Besides the woman's experience of the placental delivery, and possible differences in the amount of blood loss, there are generally no other health risks or benefits to choosing either option for delivery of the placenta. Once the placenta is out, the doctor or midwife will usually feel to make sure that your uterus is contracting and check to make sure that any bleeding is slowing right down or stopping. You will also be checked to see if you tore during the birth.

I would definitely recommend having your midwife or doctor show you the placenta and take you through what all the bits do. This has been a part of your body for the last 9 months, after all. The clinician should have a detailed look at your placenta (even if you don't want to) to make sure there are no missing parts, or any other issues that could impact on the health of you or baby. In some circumstances, it may be recommended to have the placenta looked at by a pathologist if there have been any concerns with infection, or the growth of baby during the pregnancy.

What you want to do with the placenta then is up to you. Your care provider will deal with it if you have no preference. Many people choose to take their placenta home, to bury it under a tree or flower garden, or do any number of other things.

Should I encapsulate my placenta?

If you are thinking of keeping your placenta for any reason, discuss this with your midwife or doctor prior to birth so they can store it appropriately. While there is no evidence to suggest that eating the placenta in any form provides benefits to mother or baby, many women report increased energy levels and better milk production, and believe it helps with post-partum depression.

Essentially the process goes a little like this. The placenta is picked up within a few hours of birth, dehydrated, ground up into a powdered form and placed into capsules. Encapsulation isn't cheap (anywhere between $200 and $500) and it is a good idea to do your research beforehand so you're informed as to how the capsules are prepared, including sterilisation methods.

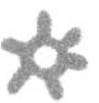

WILL I TEAR?

In some way, and at some point in your birthing career, you will most likely have a tear, even if it is only a minor one. If it is your first baby, it is more likely than not that you will tear in some way. If it is not your first baby, there is a pretty good chance that you will not tear. However, most tears from childbirth are not serious and everything usually heals up normally and quickly.

- *First-degree tears* – occur in most first births. These are usually around the opening of the vagina, but sometimes extend up the inside of the labia (inner lips of the vagina). Sometimes, the labia themselves can tear. A lot of first-degree tears do not need stitches. The reasons you may be offered stitches are if there is active bleeding, or the tear is in a position that will not sit together easily, or may be prone to rubbing when you open and close your legs.
- *Second-degree tears* – occur in at least half of first births. This is where the tear involves tissue beneath the skin, usually in the perineum. The perineum is made up of stretchy connective

tissue in the middle, with a bunch of muscles attaching and wrapping outwards around the vagina, anus and towards the inner thigh. The stuff in the middle (the perineal body) has fewer nerves and blood vessels than the stuff going out to the side. Most natural tears go roughly down the middle. For this reason, natural tears in labour do tend to bleed less and can be less painful than deliberate cuts. The perineum is basically designed to stretch and tear, but is very forgiving during healing and will heal (more or less) back to normal within a month or two of birth. For most second-degree tears, you will be offered stitches. Some tears will heal up normally without stitches, but most midwives, doctors and patients prefer to have things stitched neatly back together for added reassurance.

- *Third-degree tears* – occur in 3–5 per cent of births. These are the ones that people are generally afraid of, as a third-degree tear involves the muscles around the anus. If you have a third-degree tear (often called obstetric anal sphincter injuries, or OASIS), it will be strongly suggested you have it repaired with stitches. In most cases, it will also be suggested you have it repaired in an operating theatre, with good anaesthetic. The concern with these types of tears is that there is a possibility of the patient having problems with anal continence if it is not repaired correctly. Fortunately, if it is recognised and repaired well, most women have no concerns at all with function afterwards. It is important to have a talk with an obstetrician about what to do next time, though. It is commonly suggested that women who have third-degree tears deliver by caesarean next time around, though each situation should be assessed on its own merits, and many women can safely have a natural birth in the future if they wish.
- *Fourth-degree tears* – are *very* uncommon. In a fourth-degree tear, the tear extends from the opening of the vagina, through all the muscle of the perineum and anus, and into the lining of the rectum. Everything written above for third-degree tears applies, but there are higher risks of complications or issues in the future. After repair, women with these types of tears need to have close support from an obstetrician to watch for any signs of problems and address them early.

EPISIOTOMY

An episiotomy is when the doctor or midwife makes a cut with scissors at the opening of the vagina to let baby out. While this sounds brutal, you will usually be given an anaesthetic injection beforehand so you don't feel any pain, and the cut is only made as big as it needs to be.

There are some advantages to an episiotomy:

- It can mean that the baby gets out a lot quicker (usually in an emergency).
- The cut is made at an angle (usually to the woman's right), to avoid the muscles around the anus.
- The cut is made in a straight line, which is usually easier to stitch back together neatly.

There are disadvantages to an episiotomy:

- You will definitely need stitches.
- They can bleed more than spontaneous tears (though very bad tears will bleed more than an episiotomy).
- Some women report that healing can be more painful, because the tension is off to one side rather than symmetrical. This is somewhat dependent on the skill and technique of the person doing the stitching.

There are definitely scenarios when one should be considered:

- If you are having a forceps or vacuum delivery (see page 209), because the head crowns and delivers in only a few contractions and there is less time to allow stretching.
- If you have had a spontaneous anal injury from a natural tear during a previous birth.
- If the head is crowning for a very long time. In this situation, it is often just a matter of waiting for a natural tear. If the head has been putting pressure on the perineum for a long time it can become very swollen, so that when it does tear it can do so in many different directions, making a neat repair more challenging.
- In an emergency, when there are concerns that the baby is in trouble.

Usually, tears are repaired within an hour or so of the birth, in the birthing suite. There is no major rush to do the stitches, unless there is significant bleeding, so you should have time to enjoy those first moments with your baby and catch your breath after the birth. Most clinicians prefer to use stirrups, or foot rests, to put stitches in after birth, which can be a little confronting if you have birthed in a more natural position. Some sterile material will be put underneath your bottom, and the skin around the vagina will be wiped with an antiseptic (which is usually a bit cold). If you don't have an epidural, some injections of local anaesthetic will be needed. You should get a warning before the sting from this needle, and an experienced clinician should be able to make the whole area numb in less than 30 seconds. This should also be the worst part in terms of pain.

There are lots of different ways to put things back together, depending on the tear, but most clinicians prefer to use one running stitch. The question 'How many stitches did I get?' is common. It is probably more relevant to ask: 'How many lengths of suture did I need?' If more than one suture thread is opened, then your tear was probably a bit deeper than average. A dissolving stitch should always be used, and is often gone from your body in less than a month.

After the stitches are put in, which should only take an experienced clinician about 15 minutes or so, they will usually poke around a bit more to ensure that everything is as it should be, then check your tummy to make sure the uterus is contracted. Often you will also be warned that an anal exam might be done. This is to make sure that there is no damage to the muscles of your anus. As an added bonus at this point, it is common to give a suppository painkiller medication, to help with discomfort when the local anaesthetic wears off.

After getting stitches from childbirth, there is not much you need to do to look after them. Ideally, you should be able to forget they are there. Don't put soaps, antiseptics or chemicals in the area, just clean water. If things continue to feel better, this is a good sign. If things feel like they are getting more swollen, sorer, have come apart or have a bad smell, you should let your doctor or midwife know. Complications from stitches in the perineum, such as infection or wound breakdown, are quite uncommon.

WHAT HAPPENS IF BABY CAN'T BE PUSHED OUT?

When a woman has been pushing for a long time, it is not unusual for an obstetrician to be asked (with various amounts of cussing and abuse) to 'just pull it out'. Nine times out of 10, this is not necessary with enough patience, but maternal exhaustion, or a 'prolonged second stage', is the most common reason for an assisted birth.

As a general principle, without any evidence of a dangerous situation for mother and baby, it would be unlikely that an obstetrician would recommend an instrumental birth with any less than an hour of effective pushing from the mother. In first-time mothers, up to 2 full hours of pushing is also reasonable, but we like to see continued evidence of progress being made, particularly over the second hour.

You need to be fully dilated to be able to have your baby born by forceps or vacuum (see page 209), but there are times when it can be a toss-up with a caesarean.

FULL-DILATATION CAESAREAN

There are some circumstances where an obstetrician will not feel comfortable using a vacuum or forceps due to a possibility of trauma to you, your baby or your pelvic floor. If an attempt at vacuum or forceps delivery has failed, the fall-back will also be a caesarean There are quite a few added challenges with full-dilatation caesarean:

- The baby's head can often be quite well wedged into the pelvis, making it just as hard to get baby out the top end as the bottom. Very occasionally, another doctor or midwife will even need to push the baby back up from down below prior to the caesarean or (rarely) during the operation.
- The lower part of the uterus is stretched and soft from labour, and is more prone to tears during delivery.
- The muscle of the uterus is tired from labour and pushing, and will sometimes take longer to contract and stop bleeding after delivery.
- Because the baby's head has been exposed to the vagina (and sometimes the outside world, to some degree), more bacteria are floating around, which can contaminate the surgical scar during delivery.

All of these factors make a caesarean riskier for a woman who has already been pushing, as compared to an elective caesarean.

A full-dilatation caesarean is no walk in the park, and is one of the common reasons why a registrar on the labour ward may call in 'the boss' for help. It is reasonably common, though, and generally things do go well.

A caesarean delivery in second stage can be extremely disappointing for a woman after all the effort she has been through to get there. Some women do make it part of their birth plan to opt for caesarean delivery over vacuum or forceps in the event that they get stuck in the second stage. I would never recommend this approach as a general principle, but certainly there are cases where the decision about whether to try an instrumental birth or go straight for caesarean is a difficult one. One such circumstance is referred to as a 'trial in theatre', which means the obstetrician is not sure it will come out.

A trial in theatre is where we transfer a woman in second stage to an operating theatre, with the intention of trying to deliver baby vaginally by forceps or vacuum in the first instance. An operating theatre is not the most ideal place for a woman to push. It is brightly lit and there are usually a bunch of strangers in blue scrubs busily doing things in all corners of the room. But what an operating theatre does provide is safety. With everything (and everybody) immediately present and ready to go, your obstetrician can be prepared for any possibility with a difficult birth.

When it comes to instrumental birth, what it also means is that the obstetrician has less pressure to get the baby out vaginally at all costs, because there is the ready availability to proceed with caesarean birth within minutes if things go pear-shaped. This willingness to abandon does not mean they will not try as hard to get the baby out vaginally; it just makes it less likely that they will do so at the risk of causing any harm to you or baby, particularly if there are concerns that baby is already struggling to cope with the labour.

Shoulder dystocia

This is when the head comes out but the shoulders are stuck. It is one of a few obstetric emergencies where minutes matter. Usually, after the baby's head is born, we wait until the next contraction and with a push, or a little gentle traction, the baby's shoulders are born and the baby comes out. Shoulder dystocia is what happens if those shoulders don't come easily.

With shoulder dystocia, the shoulders of the baby get wedged in the space between your pubic bone and sacrum (deep part of your tailbone). It is a blockage of bone on bone, not the soft tissue of the pelvic floor or vagina. The blockage is deeper inside, and harder to get at for the midwife or obstetrician.

The most critical issue is that after baby's head has been born, the umbilical cord becomes compressed deeper in the pelvis and, even though the baby's face is outside, its chest is too squished to be able to inflate its lungs and breathe. This means that baby is going without new oxygen for the duration of time from birthing the head until the rest of the body is out. We know that damage to baby from lack of oxygen can start to occur from 10 minutes in this situation, or sooner if it has been a difficult labour and baby has less reserves. Shoulder dystocia can be a cause of stillbirth in labour, which is why it is treated with such urgency.

It is also possible for the baby to suffer a broken clavicle (collar bone) or humerus (upper arm bone) during delivery. From the mother's point of view, there is a higher chance of perineal tearing, as well as the possibility of pelvic bone instability or inflammation after delivery.

Shoulder dystocia itself is not too uncommon; if it happens, it can be alarming for everybody involved, but the above examples are extreme scenarios. If a mother experiences shoulder dystocia during birth, both she and her partner will usually benefit from a lot of discussion to understand events, even if everything turns out okay (which it usually does).

ASSISTED VAGINAL DELIVERY (FORCEPS AND VACUUM)

Putting a medical instrument on the head of an unborn baby remains one of the most terrifying things that I do in my specialist practice, even after delivering hundreds of babies this way. However, serious complications are very uncommon in experienced hands. Without the potential to help a woman and baby make it through a difficult vaginal delivery, the art of obstetrics would be a shadow of what it is. A well done instrumental birth can certainly still maintain the calm and magic of a spontaneous vaginal birth and, in the right circumstances, an assisted birth can make a very positive difference to the outcome for both mother and baby.

Depending on the hospital and practitioner, an assisted vaginal delivery may be performed in between 1 in 10 to 1 in 7 labours in Australian hospitals. There are a number of reasons why assisted birth may be offered:

- Prolonged second stage – if a woman has been pushing for a long time, there are increased risks both for mother and baby. This may lead to a recommendation for assisted birth after 2 hours in first labours, or after 1 hour in people who have had a vaginal birth previously.
- Maternal exhaustion – the decision may be made a little earlier if the mother has requested assistance, or clearly needs help.
- Fetal distress – when there is a concern about the wellbeing of the baby, usually due to a non-reassuring change in the pattern of the heartbeat during the pushing part. A lot of these births can be quite straightforward mechanically, as there is often nothing to suggest that the baby is too big, the mother's pelvis too small, or the head facing the wrong way. The biggest concern with this reason for an assisted birth is controlling the adrenaline in the room. When there is concern about the heartbeat of the baby, it is easy for emotions to take over, both for the parents, and also for the doctor.
- Medical issues for the women that may make it dangerous for her to push extremely hard (such as some heart conditions).

There are two main types of tools that we use to help get babies out vaginally: vacuum (ventouse) and forceps. Ultimately, the judgement regarding which instrument is the right tool for the job will come down to the obstetrician.

There are important things to consider before an assisted vaginal delivery is performed:

- Is the mother fully dilated? An instrumental birth should (generally) never be done if there is still cervix hanging around, as this has a higher chance of injuring the mother, and the baby is not likely to come out. Besides the cervix being fully dilated, the obstetrician should also be confident the baby's head is low enough in the vagina to make an assisted birth safe. If there are any doubts, they may consider a trial in theatre (see page 207).
- Does the mother (and her partner) understand what is about to happen, why it is recommended and the potential for complications? This is called informed consent, and while it does not require a written signature in this circumstance, if somebody is about to put something inside your vagina and onto your baby's head, you probably want an idea of why they are doing it and what could potentially happen.
- What is the plan for pain relief? If there is a working epidural, no worries. If not, your obstetrician should have a word with you about other methods to make you numb down there, as it will likely be a bit more intense than a spontaneous birth.
- Is the bladder empty? You may think you have done plenty of wees during the labour, but when a baby's head is squishing your bladder and urethra, your bladder may be much fuller than you think. When we are about to navigate a really tight fit getting that head out, the more space the better. If your bladder is full, pulling on the baby (and hence on your bladder) may also be bad news for your future pelvic floor function. For this reason, the doctor should generally use a catheter to empty your bladder completely before putting anything else inside the vagina.

A lot of babies that are being helped out are getting help for a reason: either they have had a long hard labour, with a lot of pushing, or there are changes in their heart rate pattern that are concerning. Either way, there is a good chance that the baby may be exhausted and need a little perking up. A paediatric doctor will usually be present for this reason.

Vacuum delivery

The most commonly used devices in Australian hospitals are handheld, with a disc shape 6–7 cm in diameter. (The bell-shaped cups are less commonly used.) The vacuum cup is put on the top of baby's head in the optimal position that we want to be leading through the birth canal (called the flexion point). When we pull down, it is still very important for the mother to push hard. I tell mothers that, when I am using the vacuum, I am steering the baby in the right direction, but they are still the engine providing the power. Typically, baby is delivered in around three contractions when a vacuum is used, but it can take a few more.

When the doctor puts the vacuum device on, they create a suction between the cup of the vacuum and the skin on the baby's scalp. This suction will leave a bruise on baby's skin, a bit like a hickey ('love bite'), which will take a few days to disappear. It will also cause an exaggerated swelling of fluid under the skin called a chignon, which is usually gone within the first 15 minutes. Occasionally, it can cause heavier bleeding under the scalp, which will require observation and can occasionally be problematic.

This type of birth is often seen as a gentle way to help deliver a baby but that reputation is probably more applicable to the mother than the baby. The vacuum is also more likely to fail when used to achieve a vaginal birth, meaning that either the forceps are then used for a second attempt, or the mother ends up with a caesarean.

The vacuum cups are designed to pop off if the baby is not coming, or the doctor is pulling too hard. When it happens, it can be quite dramatic. There is a sound like a bottle of champagne being opened, and the doctor may stumble backwards. I have seen many soon-to-be-dads go as white as ghosts when this happens.

Forceps delivery

Although forceps have a poorer public reputation than suction cups, they can actually be a little gentler on the baby (when used in the right way at the right time). The forceps wrap around the entirety of the baby's head rather than just pulling on the scalp. This allows the obstetrician a greater degree of control over how fast or slow the birth is, and distributes the force more evenly around baby's head. However, the use of forceps means the mother is more likely to need an episiotomy. It is also trickier to use them comfortably for the woman without an epidural.

The forceps are more likely to achieve a vaginal birth than the vacuum, and are less reliant on the mother being able to push strongly and effectively, though pushing hard is still the most important thing that a woman can do to help get the baby out quickly and safely with an assisted birth. It can leave some bruising marks around the cheeks or the side of the baby's head. More significant injuries to babies from forceps are very uncommon.

In my experience, a lot of women are less fearful of the idea of forceps (some even say they prefer the idea to vacuum) when it is discussed antenatally. While nobody puts an instrumental birth at the top of their wish list, it is something that any woman planning a vaginal birth should have a little bit of preparation for, to make the idea less frightening if it happens.

WHAT HAPPENS IF I BLEED AFTER THE BIRTH?

There is usually some blood loss after birth. Some women lose very little, but the average loss is generally about 200–300 ml. Any blood loss more than 500 ml after birth is regarded as abnormal, and referred to as a post-partum haemorrhage (PPH). When you are pregnant, the amount of blood your body is able to pump through the uterus and placenta is around 1 litre per minute. In theory, this means that your entire blood volume passes through the uterus every 5 to 10 minutes. That is how quickly it is possible to have life-threatening blood loss after birth. However, most PPHs are somewhat slower than this and don't usually progress to be life threatening. The chance of having more than 1 litre blood loss after birth is around 1 in 100.

If your bleeding becomes excessive, you doctor or midwife might:

- Get the placenta out, if it isn't out already.
- Put their hand firmly on the fundus of your uterus and very firmly press down into your tummy. This is to keep the muscle of the uterus contracted and stop it from leaking further blood.
- Put in an intravenous saline drip and a catheter. By keeping your bladder empty, the uterus is able to shrink down further, which helps to stop further blood loss.
- Give medication to help the uterus contract more strongly. These drugs are collectively called uterotonics, and may be given through an intravenous line or as an injection. Some medication can be given as a suppository, which is better and more quickly absorbed than through your stomach.
- Check your vagina for bleeding directly from a tear.

If you are still bleeding after all of this, it may be suggested you be transferred to an operating theatre. This can be very disappointing as it means being separated from your baby, and often having a general anaesthetic or an epidural, if one hasn't already been used. In most cases, the main reasons to use an operating theatre are to look for tears in the vagina or cervix that are bleeding, and to feel inside the uterus for leftover placenta, which might be contributing to the bleeding. Occasionally, a sterile balloon is placed inside the uterus and filled with fluid to put pressure on blood vessels from the inside. Sometimes, sterile gauze is packed in the vagina to add pressure.

After a PPH, you will need to be watched very closely. If you have a very low blood count the next day, or experience a lot of dizziness or breathlessness, a blood transfusion will be offered. The amount of blood loss required to need a blood transfusion is usually pretty high (around 1.5 litres in women who were not low to begin with). The highest risk for bleeding after birth is usually in the first 4–6 hours, but delayed bleeding can occur even days after birth. It is always important to talk with your doctor or midwife about what level of bleeding to expect when you go home, and if you are ever worried about the amount of bleeding, get seen sooner rather than later. As a rough guide, if the bleeding is worse than the heaviest day of your period and is bright red, it is more likely to be abnormal.

CAESAREAN BIRTH

When it comes to birth, there are few issues more polarising than the C-section. This is when the baby bypasses the vagina and comes out through a cut in the tummy. Opinions on caesarean birth vary widely between obstetricians, midwives and pregnant women. There are some women who enter a pregnancy with no intention of going through a natural birth. There are other women who feel that a caesarean birth is the worst outcome imaginable. I am not going to enter a debate about which group is right. The purpose of what you are about to read is to make you prepared for a caesarean birth if it occurs, for whatever reason.

In general, there are two main types of caesarean birth, emergency and elective. These terms are a bit misleading, because an elective caesarean may well be for a reason out of the woman's control, and possibly something they are not really electing to have. It more correctly means that the caesarean has been planned in advance, usually for a medical indication. Similarly, an emergency caesarean may not be lights-and-sirens stuff (although it can be). Emergency caesareans are those that are done during labour, usually for reasons that have emerged during the course of labour.

In Australia, the most common reasons for caesarean birth are:

Elective caesarean

- The woman has had one or more previous caesarean births.
- The baby is presenting breech at term.
- The placenta is too low to safely attempt labour.
- The doctor feels that baby is too big to attempt vaginal birth.
- Previous vaginal birth has resulted in significant injury to mother or baby. The most common example of this is a prior anal sphincter injury, although for a lot of women, vaginal birth is still a safe option. Another common reason is a history of shoulder dystocia.
- Other medical risk factors may make vaginal birth unsafe.
- Maternal request – when there is no strict medical indication for the baby to be born by caesarean. This is the least common reason for caesarean birth in most Australian hospitals. In the situation where a caesarean is the mother's preference, detailed

discussions should occur between the woman and obstetrician to try to understand the reasons for this choice. Many times, with a plan of action to address any concerns, women may try a natural birth with reassurance that caesarean is available.

Emergency caesarean

- There is a suspicion that the baby has become distressed.
- 'Failure to progress' – this phrase applies to a situation where the cervix has stopped dilating, and the baby is not getting closer to being born. It is a terrible description. The word 'failure' should never be applied to a description of birth. Another is 'obstructed labour', although certainly there are times when things seem to stop, despite there being no suggestion of an obstruction.
- Failed instrumental – where an attempt has been made at forceps or vacuum delivery, but the obstetrician has abandoned further attempts due to a concern for mother or baby's safety.
- Sudden and severe medical conditions arising during the labour for the mother (such as an eclamptic seizure).
- 'Malpresentation' – which means the baby is trying to come through the cervix in a way that is not safe to continue with a vaginal birth. The most common reason is a breech presentation discovered in labour, where the doctor or patient is not confident to proceed. Other situations likely to require a caesarean in labour include the baby coming out face first, or a hand or foot coming down. Also included is the umbilical cord coming first (cord presentation or cord prolapse). A much more likely position for the baby, which is a common reason for caesarean, is if the baby is in an occipitoposterior presentation. While it is not dangerous for baby to come down looking face up, it does make labour more difficult. Often posterior presentations go hand in hand with stalled labour. Most occipitoposterior babies will still be able to be delivered vaginally, just not necessarily with the easiest labour or delivery.
- The most dramatic situation is called a 'crash' (or category 1) caesarean. This is where we drop everything and push the bed to an operating theatre without any delay due to a life-threatening emergency. In this circumstance, often the mother is required to be put to sleep and partners may not be allowed to attend the birth.

PREPARING FOR CAESAREAN DELIVERY

The following is a very broad generalisation of the experience that many women have if they are advised to go through with a caesarean delivery during the course of their labour, where there is no immediate concern for the safety of baby or mother.

Keep in mind there can be quite a few things that change depending on the obstetrician, the hospital and certain circumstances for the woman or baby.

- **Consent.** Once the initial discussion with the doctor has occurred, and the woman has agreed to undergo caesarean delivery, the doctor will then need to obtain legal written consent to perform the surgery. This means that you sign a piece of paper agreeing that you understand the reason for the procedure, the possible risks, any alternatives that are available and that you give permission to proceed. The doctor will need to mention that there is a possibility of complications and what these could be. Broadly speaking, the complications of caesarean birth include a risk of infection during surgical healing, a small chance of damage to nearby organs including the bladder and bowel and an increased chance of excessive bleeding, including a decision about the acceptability of blood transfusion if this became life-threatening. The doctor may also mention the implications of a caesarean birth on your postnatal recovery and any future pregnancy, as a caesarean delivery may increase the likelihood of caesarean birth being required for future children. The moment of signing on the dotted line can be an emotional moment for women and their partners, particularly after a long and exhausting labour.
- **Transfer to theatre.** The midwives and/or nurses will make sure you are changed into a hospital-issue gown and hairnet. You will be asked to remove any underwear. Partners will get changed into scrubs and matching hairnet (they do get to keep their underwear on). A wardsperson may come into the labour room to push your bed to the operating theatre, or else you will be moved onto another bed in preparation. You will then be wheeled down the corridor and/or into the elevator, to the door of the theatre. On entering the theatre complex, you will be greeted by a world of

people in coloured hats and scrubs. You will be asked a checklist of questions, including when you last ate and drank, any allergies, dental work (in case you need a breathing tube in an emergency) and, before you are allowed to enter the theatre, generally you will be asked to say in your own words what you are having done. You will also be given a shot of a solution to drink, to neutralise acid in your stomach, in case you need a breathing tube or become nauseous when you are lying flat in the operating theatre.

- **The partner gets to wait outside.** This can be an anxious time. Most hospitals will ask the support person (such as the partner) to wait outside while arrangements are made with the anaesthetic and getting the patient prepared. This can take half an hour, often longer. By the time they are ushered into the theatre, it is usually 'go time', and the baby is often out within a few minutes. It is not unusual to see couples shed a few tears when they temporarily get separated at the doors of the operating theatre.
- **The anaesthetist will do their thing.** Once again, you may be quick-fired a list of questions about your health and any risks. If you do not have an epidural, they will talk you through the process of giving one (or more commonly a variation on this called a 'spinal anaesthetic', which is not as long-lasting, but gives denser numbness). If you already have an epidural, they will usually need to top it up with more drugs, to make sure that you are extra numb. This epidural top-up can sometimes cause your blood pressure to drop, which could cause nausea and can have an effect on baby's heart rate. The midwife will check on the heart during this process to make sure that baby is happy. Occasionally, if these drugs overshoot the mark, you can start to feel numb too high on the chest and possibly this can make you feel anxious or have difficulty breathing. The anaesthetist will continually check the sensation on your skin with an ice cube and ask if it feels cold. This is because the same nerves that carry temperature sensation are involved in pain signals. Once the anaesthetist is happy that you have an effective epidural or spinal, you will be transferred to the operating table.

- **The operating table.** Being on the operating table before your baby is born can make you feel extremely vulnerable. You are awake, in a strange place, with strangers all around your body, which is variously exposed. It is not unusual for eight or more people to be in an operating theatre preparing for a caesarean birth. There are typically three nurses, a midwife, a paediatrician, the anaesthetist, the obstetrician, the obstetrician's assistant and a wardsperson, as well as any trainee doctors or various professional students (especially in a public hospital) who may be learning from the other staff. This can be quite a shock for the unprepared couple. You will also need a catheter in your bladder. This may have already been inserted in the labour ward (particularly if you had an epidural earlier). If it hasn't been put in earlier, this will need to put in, which can also be a confronting thing to have done in such a busy environment. A good obstetrician will generally try to be discreet about this, and protect your modesty as much as possible. You may also need to have some pubic hair shaved off above your pubic bone. Once everything is prepared, the nurse and obstetrician will paint your tummy, groin and upper thighs with antiseptic, and put some sterile sheets over everything except the lower half of your belly. This will be lifted like a curtain in front of you so that you can't see what is going on over the other side. At this point, your support person is generally allowed to come inside and will get a seat by your side at the head of the bed.
- **Starting the surgery.** Before starting the surgery, the obstetrician will communicate with the anaesthetist to make sure that you are numb enough to proceed. They will often pinch your skin in a few places under the belly button and the anaesthetist will check to make sure you don't feel anything sharp or pointy. It is common to feel pressure, or know you are being touched, but not to feel pain or sharpness. After this check, the obstetrician will proceed.

WHAT TO EXPECT DURING A CAESAREAN

- A cut is made above the pubic bone, usually about 2–3 cm above the bone, often a bit higher. The cut will need to be long enough to get baby's head out (10–12 cm), but may be a little longer, depending on the experience of your obstetrician and any factors that make it important to have extra space. The cut may have a slight curve but can be straight, depending on how high it is and the width of your pelvis. Very occasionally, an obstetrician will make a vertical cut between pubic bone and belly button, but this is only for complicated situations, and you should have been informed if this is going to happen.
- There are a few layers to get through to get to baby. All people have a layer of fatty tissue, followed by a white sheet of collagen around the muscles (the rectus sheath), both of which are cut in the same direction as the skin. The muscles are not cut, but stretched apart at the natural gap in the middle. This can often be felt, and you may get a warning to feel a stretch. The next layer is a filmy, thin layer inside the abdominal cavity called peritoneum, which is often stretched with the muscle. The obstetrician will now be able to see the uterus. There is another layer of peritoneum over the surface of the uterus and bladder. This will be opened to make sure that your bladder can be tucked safely out of the way. At this point, you will often be told that baby is about to be born.
- Your support person may be scrambling to turn on their camera. A lot of hospitals will allow still photography during a caesarean birth, but you will usually need special permission if you're hoping to get some video. There may be somebody there who will help out by taking the photos to allow both you and your support person to focus on the birth (there sure will be enough people in the room). A lot of couples don't want any photos at all, which is okay as well. Meanwhile, the obstetrician will make a very careful incision across the bottom of your uterus and break your waters. You will hear a sloshing and gurgling sound as the amniotic fluid is sucked into a canister. The obstetrician will put their hand into your womb and under the baby's head. Often, they may also use a pair of obstetric forceps to hold the baby's head.

- You will often get a warning that you are 'going to feel a lot of pushing'. The obstetrician's assistant will be pressing down firmly on the top of your uterus, under your ribs. This is to push the baby out, while the obstetrician directs the head out towards the skin with their hand or forceps. Once the baby's head is out, the obstetrician will need to bring out the shoulders, then the baby will be born. The cord will generally be cut on the sterile area of the drape. At some point, the curtain may be lowered so you can see your baby, and find out the gender, if you didn't already know.
- A midwife will receive the baby and often the baby will be immediately taken over to a small bed to be woken up, warmed and dried with a towel. It may also need to be given a little oxygen, which is not always a sign there is anything wrong, so don't be too concerned. On that note, you might not be able to see too much during the first few minutes after the birth, as you will still be flat on your back and the curtain will be pulled back up. Support persons are usually allowed to walk over to the bed with the baby and watch what is happening, and touch the baby. Some women may feel better having their support person by their side, though. If your baby is doing well, you will be able to hold them while the surgery is being completed. This can often be quite awkward, as there is not a lot of space under the sterile curtain and often the baby is too close to your face, or your arms are tied up with drips and blood pressure cuffs. It is also common for women to start to feel nauseous after the baby is out. You may need to vomit, which can be a very hard thing to do lying on your back. With a bit of warning though, there are sick bags, and the anaesthetist will be able to give medication to help with nausea and improve your blood pressure.
- Meanwhile, the obstetrician will be delivering your placenta. This will also be kept for the midwife to check, and whatever destiny the placenta originally had can be fulfilled. After the placenta is out, the obstetrician will clean the inside of the uterus and make sure there is no tissue left behind. For this reason, women commonly stop bleeding more quickly than they do after a natural birth. The doctors will now have to close the hole they have made in your abdomen, starting with the uterus. It is unavoidable for there to be bleeding at this point. This can often look a bit shocking

if you or your partner catch a glimpse of the drapes or the suction canister. It is not unusual to lose up to 500 ml of blood (compared with around 300 ml during a natural birth). The bleeding usually stops when the obstetrician has finished closing the uterus. All the stitches used inside your body are made of a substance that is absorbed over time, so nothing on the inside will be permanent or need to be removed down the track.

- Once the uterus is closed, the obstetrician will check for any other points of bleeding and sweep out some of the fluid and clots from inside your abdomen. They will usually check your tubes and ovaries while they are there, to make sure they are healthy. I've heard the experience described as feeling 'like they are doing the washing up inside your tummy' or 'rummaging in a handbag'. It may be a relatively close description of what you might feel but doesn't make it sound any more appealing than what is actually going on.
- On the way out, the obstetrician will need to close the layers that were opened getting in. This is very straightforward, as all the stitching is in straight lines. During training, a caesarean is often one of the first procedures that registrars or even more junior doctors learn how to do. In some ways, closing a caesarean is easier than putting together the vagina after a tricky tear, which often has ragged edges. The main part you are going to see is the skin, though, so this is where the variation comes in. Most obstetricians use a dissolving stitch threaded just under the skin so there is nothing to see but a thin line on the skin. Some use a long stitch that is pulled out after a week. In certain cases, metal skin staples may be used, which need to be removed later on. There are various arguments about which technique leaves less noticeable scars. I think the reality is more to do with each woman's genetics (some people are prone to scarring), how carefully the skin is put together and how well the wound is cared for in the weeks after.
- Once the surgery is completed, the nurse will clean off all the antiseptic (especially if it is the brown iodine). The doctor will usually press on the top of your womb, which should now be down at the level of your belly button, and try to squeeze any clots out that may have formed. This is much more comfortable to do while you are still numb, compared with when the epidural wears

off, but nonetheless can be a bit unpleasant. They may put a swab in the vagina to help sweep out the clots. Baby will often go with the midwife and support person to the recovery area while you are being cleaned up. You will need to be in the operating theatre recovery area for up to an hour, just to be watched for immediate post-operative complications.

- Most hospitals try to accommodate keeping the baby with mother at all times, but it is worth knowing that there are occasions when a mother may be separated from her baby for an hour or more after the birth. Obviously, if the baby is stressed or otherwise unwell from the labour, there are times when this is unavoidable as some babies will need support from the nursery doctors. Sometimes, though, if the hospital can't spare a midwife to stay with you and baby in recovery, then a perfectly well baby might be taken to the nursery to be watched until you are returned to the maternity ward. Most hospitals make efforts to avoid this kind of disruption to those initial bonding moments. In the majority of cases, your baby will be with you the whole time and many women are able to have the baby attach to the breast and have their first feed during this time.

What I'm really thinking:

Caesarean birth

To be honest, I was most nervous about the spinal. I was asked to lean over while the anaesthetist pressed on different areas of my spine. It didn't hurt when the needle went in – I just experienced a sharp sensation (like having a blood test) that quickly subsided. But I was shaking the entire time! A few moments later, I felt a warm sensation through my legs as they became numb. I was rolled onto the surgical table and a catheter was inserted in my bladder so I didn't have to worry about going to the toilet for the next day or so.

I had all the cords placed on one arm so that I could have my robe slightly off and one arm free for when my baby was born. This allowed for immediate skin-to-skin contact, which was an important part of my birth plan.

The obstetrician then began touching around my abdomen asking if I could feel anything. And then after what felt like 15 minutes of pulling and tugging, none of which was painful but not overly comfortable either, I heard the first cry.

The curtain dropped, and I saw my baby in full view for the first time. It was intense and overwhelming, yet so magical. What felt like a crowded room full of people just vanished: it was just me, my partner and this tiny new being that I had loved deeply for the past 9 months. My partner was given the option to cut the cord and as the medical team continued to work around me, time seemed to go so quickly; in fact, so quickly, I cannot even remember it – I was just consumed by my baby, caught up in the moment, filled with absolute joy and contentment. The midwife checked over my baby to make sure all was well and then placed her immediately on my chest for her very first feed.

MAKING CAESAREAN A BIRTH, NOT JUST A SURGERY

A caesarean is a surgical procedure. It is also a birth.

That might sound like an obvious statement, but it took me a few years into my training to recognise how sidelined the birth part of a caesarean can be.

Some doctors would boast about how quickly they could do a caesarean, or how small they could make their incision. Nobody seemed to talk about the experience for the woman, or how discreetly the operator could perform a caesarean. I think it is something that only comes with time and attending hundreds of births. The births that are the most wonderful are not necessarily the cleanest or the most perfect. They are the ones in which there are the fewest distractions, where everything is there to make the birth safe, but it is not *in the way*; those moments when new parents are able to reach out and take their baby and everything else just happens, without disturbing the bubble of that moment.

Caesarean birth is becoming more acceptable and safer all the time. There are even strong arguments for how caesarean may be beneficial for certain elements of future pelvic floor health. What we can still do much better is to keep that focus on the birth and try to avoid disturbing that bubble of time when mother and baby meet each other face to face for the first time.

Below are some of the things that women having a caesarean can talk to their obstetrician about in order to preserve that moment as much as is safe and feasible in an operating room environment.

Setting the mood. An operating theatre is a loud, bright and complicated space, with a lot going on. This can be a very nerve-wracking place for a couple to be in. It is also probably not the best introduction to the world for a newborn baby. Of course, it also needs to be a safe space for the staff involved in doing the procedure to do their job. With some planning, and permission from relevant staff in the operating facility, there are a number of ways that this environment can be more conducive to birth. It may be possible to have the room lights dimmed, making it more comfortable for baby to open their eyes. A lot of obstetricians will be happy to have some music playing in the room and may let you bring your own (as long as it is appropriately calming). The most important aspect, however, is the other people in the room. Sometimes it can feel like ring-leading a circus, but a good obstetrician should try to encourage a calm, peaceful and respectful environment. It is very easy for theatre staff to be going about their business, chatting and talking amongst themselves. Generally, when it comes to the actual birth, mostly people are quiet, but before and after it can sometimes feel like a party.

Watch the birth. Not the surgery. I don't think anyone wants to see themselves being cut open and their innards fiddled with. This goes for partners as well. But watch the birth. A lot of obstetricians are happy to drop the drapes when the baby is fully delivered. A lot of them will also be happy to drop the curtain before the head is fully out, so that the parents can watch their child emerge from the womb, and see the eyes opening and that first gasp of air as they spring into life. It will usually not be too confronting, and for those moments you won't see any blood and guts. For the woman, this can be better facilitated by elevating the shoulders either by lifting the back of the bed, or using a pillow.

Ask to have your baby ASAP. With most natural births, the baby is immediately brought up for the mother to hold. Some women, or partners, even like to take the baby immediately from between the legs and bring baby up to their chest and faces with their own hands. In a typical caesarean birth, this is usually not the case. Mostly, the baby is quickly flashed to the parents and taken across the room for a freshen up. Of course, limited delays are often vital when there is a safety concern, such as the presence of meconium in the waters around the baby. When a baby is in good condition, it is possible to give baby immediately to the mother. It is important that the area around the operation is kept sterile, but with a little planning, I generally try to put the baby straight onto the mother's chest within the first few moments of birth. With this approach, it is also possible to delay the umbilical cord clamping, if this is important to the couple. The main goal is to allow skin-to-skin contact between the mother and baby, which is recognised as an important aspect of maternal bonding and the physiology of breastfeeding for baby.

AFTER THE CAESAREAN

After caesarean birth, all the normal postnatal stuff applies. You will also be recovering from abdominal surgery, so expect to be sore. You will need to stay in hospital a bit longer than you might after a vaginal birth (at least a couple of nights). The doctors and midwives will also need to keep a close eye on you in the first 2 days for operative complications, such as ongoing bleeding or fever. You will have the catheter in your bladder at least until you are able to move your legs to get up and about, but on average, it will stay in for the first night. Your abdomen will be a bit more distended than after a vaginal birth, as the bowels often go on strike after open surgery. People will also be more interested in whether or not you are passing wind (a good sign that things are normalising inside).

It is more likely that you will require strong pain relief after a caesarean birth. Some women are concerned about taking prescription painkillers with breastfeeding. There are no major concerns about the small amount of these medications that may be present in breastmilk, and trying to be tough without the drugs is probably more likely to impact your feeding, due to the body's physiological responses to pain. By the time breastmilk fully comes in (day 3 or 4), a lot of women will be off the strong stuff altogether.

Your obstetrician will give you some advice about looking after the wound from the caesarean, depending on their technique and preferences for closing the skin. As a general principle, you should try to look at the wound at least once a day (or have somebody else have a look if it is difficult to see). Complications of wound healing, such as infection, often don't become obvious until 4 or more days after the operation, when you will likely be out of the hospital and focused on your new baby. Increasing pain, redness, wetness or separation of the skin are generally signs that you should get the wound checked again by a doctor. We don't tend to give antibiotics routinely after the caesarean (unless there has already been a concern for infection), but if antibiotics are needed, they are very likely safe to breastfeed with and most commonly are the same drugs used to treat mastitis.

Vaginal bleeding after caesarean is often a lot lighter and resolves more quickly than it does after a vaginal birth. To some degree, this is due to the fact that the placenta and membranes from the pregnancy are more easily able to be completely cleared from the womb after a caesarean. In the first day after the birth, doctors or midwives may frequently feel for the top of your uterus (usually around the belly button) to make sure that there is no blood pooling within the womb.

In the first 6 weeks, you will need to be a little more cautious about using your abdominal muscles for things like lifting, which can be especially tricky if you have other small children who are used to being carried around. Ease into things gently over this time, and the first time you do things that are a little more strenuous, take it easy until you know your muscles can handle it.

Your doctor should also have a talk to you about 'next time'. This is covered on page 251, but a discussion about the events around your particular birth and things that may be important for the next pregnancy is often helpful around the time of the birth itself, especially as next time you may have a different doctor, or be in an entirely different hospital, where accurate knowledge about the events around your birth (and the reasons for a caesarean) may not be easily attainable. This discussion is often referred to as a debriefing.

Injections after C-section

Heparin injections are given to women after C-section births to prevent clots in the legs, known as deep vein thrombosis (DVT). The injections are given into the leg or the stomach. Each woman is different as to how long they will have to have the injections. You may be sent home with the injections and asked to give them to yourself (or your partner can) for a number of days after the birth.

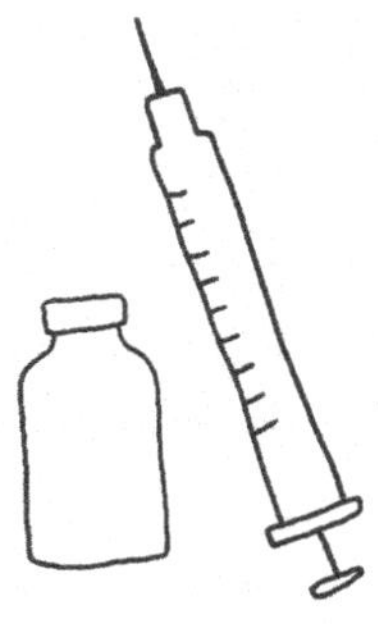

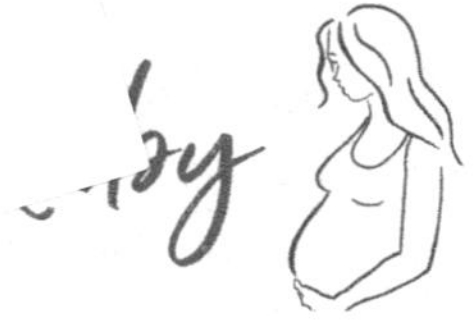

Recovering from caesarean

I have to be honest: the first few days after my caesarean were not the easiest. Dealing with the pain (and the fear of looking at the incision!) and trying to get comfortable were the hardest aspects. But giving myself plenty of time to heal and asking for help when I needed it allowed me to rest and recover.

The recovery time for caesarean tends to be longer than that for a vaginal birth. You will be given regular medication to help alleviate the pain: it's really important to keep on top of this. There may be some itching and swelling around your incision site as it heals. This can be a normal part of the healing process, but if you have any concerns, consult your doctor. Wearing loose-fitting clothing for a few weeks and choosing underwear that isn't restrictive will help to make you feel more comfortable and avoid irritation to the area.

When you go to the toilet, or sneeze or laugh, holding your stomach around the incision can help to alleviate discomfort, especially in the first couple of weeks when it is most sensitive and sore. If you're breastfeeding, propping a pillow over your stomach and placing baby on the pillow can help you to sit up straight and relieve pressure on the incision.

Your doctor or midwife will tell you when to remove the tape that covers your incision. The first time I did this it was quite painful, mostly because pubic hair grows underneath the tape and it is like getting a wax, not to mention the soreness and tenderness of the actual incision. I wouldn't suggest ripping it off like a bandaid; there are wipes that can help remove and loosen the adhesive side of the tape.

You will also wear compression stockings to prevent clotting after surgery. Doctors recommend you wear them for a few weeks. Many health professionals say to avoid driving for up to 6 weeks. You may also want to check with your car insurer to see what your policy states.

David

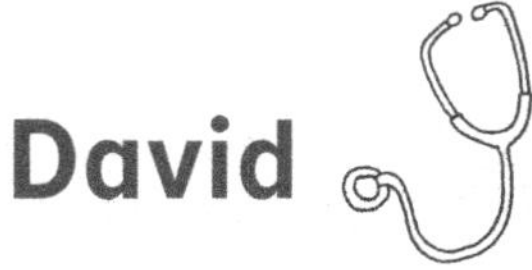

NBAC – NEXT BIRTH AFTER CAESAREAN

When a woman is pregnant after having had one or more babies previously delivered by caesarean, the medical term is NBAC. One caesarean does not necessarily mean that is the way all future babies will need to come. When an attempt is made at vaginal birth in the future, it is called a VBAC – vaginal birth after caesarean. There are a few added risks in a future pregnancy when there has been a previous caesarean. There is an area on the front of the uterus where the muscle has been opened and will have been replaced with collagen during healing. Most of the time, this is a side-to-side cut, but occasionally will be up and down (classical caesarean). The shape of the scar on the skin is not always the same as the direction of the cut on the uterus either.

The uterus is a large muscle shaped like a funnel. The muscle fibres are arranged in a spiral pattern towards the cervix, which means when the muscle squeezes (during a contraction), whatever is in the uterus is pushed down towards the neck of the funnel. The muscle is strongest at the top and gets thinner towards the cervix, where the muscle is gradually replaced with stretchy collagen. This junction between the muscle and cervix is called the lower segment. As long as the obstetrician has made their cut in this segment, usually not too much of the muscle has been cut, and the direction of the cut runs more or less parallel to the muscle fibres in the spiral. With this sort of cut, future muscle contractions will pull in the same direction as the scar. If the cut goes upwards, it moves into thicker muscle, and the cut is against the grain of the muscle, which means if the muscle contracts in future it will pull directly against the scar.

Other things that can have an impact on how the wall of the uterus heals include how many previous times it has been cut (the number of previous caesareans) and any complications during the surgery or healing period, such as infection. In summary, after a woman has had a caesarean, there is a point of potential weakness in the uterus. For this reason, any attempt at natural labour needs to be treated with a little more caution than another birth without this issue.

The most dramatic complication is uterine rupture, which basically means the previous scar starts to tear inside. This is quite uncommon, often quoted as a 1 in 200 risk for woman with a single uncomplicated caesarean in the past. This is not the risk of mother and baby dying. This is the risk of all complications related to scar tearing, from minor to life threatening. When compared to all the risks inherent in a caesarean itself, some would even argue that natural labour is at least as safe an option as an elective repeat caesarean birth.

Most hospitals in Australia will offer women a choice of how they want to give birth with their NBAC. There are some areas of the country where policy shift is quite focused on increasing women's awareness and uptake of vaginal birth after caesarean, to the point where the choice may not be given to women for method of birth. Speak with your care providers about your own particular circumstances if you are unsure about how to have your baby after a previous caesarean. One of the most common reasons for women worrying about a repeat attempt at labour and natural birth is a fear of having a caesarean anyway. In a well-supported unit, women can have a 60–70 per cent success rate for achieving natural birth with NBAC.

For the 1 out of 3 women who has a caesarean during labour, there are also lots of benefits to having 'given it a go'. Hormonally, mother and baby are better prepared for the postnatal period when they have both been through the hormonal transition of labour. Babies are more likely to have a strong cry and breathe on their own following in-labour caesarean, as having had the waters break and the uterus contract allows the fluid to be squeezed out of the baby's lungs ready for the first breath. Breastmilk also seems to come in stronger and earlier for women who have experienced labour, compared with cold caesarean. There is also the psychological advantage of having tried, and not forever wondering 'what if'.

Some women feel that, emotionally, they would frame a caesarean during repeat labour as a failure. This concept could not be further from the truth. If a woman is concerned about 'failing' at a VBAC, I try to talk to them about reframing those thoughts as 'succeeding at labour'. Labour is its own achievement. Vaginal birth is a second achievement, and both are valuable in their own way. I even come across patients who are not able to have a vaginal birth (for various medical reasons) who have a goal to at least experience labour.

HAVING TWINS

While it is possible to carry more than two babies inside the uterus, twins are by far the most common. Most people know of two types of twins: identical twins and fraternal (non-identical) twins. The first type share the same pattern of chromosomes (DNA) because they originally came from one fertilised egg that split into two. The second type are born from two separate fertilised eggs, and have a different combination of the parents' DNA, so they are like normal siblings who happened to share the womb at the same time. For this reason, fraternal twins can be opposite genders, whereas identical twins will always be the same gender.

To the obstetrician, the more important distinction between types of twins comes down to two main issues:

1. Do they share the same placenta?
2. Do they share the same bag of waters (amniotic sac)?

All fraternal twins will have their own separate placenta and amniotic sac. Most identical twins will share a placenta, and fewer will share an amniotic sac. However, some identical twins can have completely separate placentas and amniotic sacs, too. Basically, if they are different genders, you can be sure they are not identical. Otherwise, unless they share a placenta, you will usually have to wait until they come out to know for sure if they are identical or not.

Twin pregnancies with two placentas and two amniotic sacs are called diamniotic/dichorionic pregnancies (DCDA). These are the most common types of twins. If the placenta is shared but there are two sacs, we call it monochorionic/diamniotic (MCDA). If both the placenta and the bag of waters are shared, this is called monochorionic/monoamniotic (MCMA). This last type is the least common type of twin pregnancy (apart from conjoined twins). To the obstetrician, the pattern of how the placentas and sac are shared or separate is of more relevance than whether or not they are identical, because this will have the most impact on how the pregnancy is monitored for any problems. Sharing a placenta or amniotic sac poses additional challenges, which will be discussed separately.

WHEN THERE ARE TWO PLACENTAS (DCDA)

When there is twice as much placenta, there is twice as much potential for the placenta to have an effect on you. In particular, concerns like high blood pressure or high blood sugar levels are thought to be more common with twin pregnancy. As these are routinely screened for, they will usually become apparent if they become an issue.

Growth of twins can be hard to keep track of just by feeling your tummy and using a tape measure. You might be getting bigger, but how can we know that both babies are getting an even share? It is very common for fraternal twins to be different sizes. What is more important is that we don't miss one baby who has slowed or stopped growing, which is more common with twins than in single-baby pregnancies. Each placenta has its own implantation site in the womb and sometimes one site could be more fertile ground. When one twin has slowed down its growth compared to the other, we call it discordant growth. This situation poses the same questions as a single baby who is not growing enough, mainly about deciding if early delivery is needed (see page 143). With twins, however, it may happen a bit earlier, and the decisions become harder the earlier in a pregnancy you have to make them.

To monitor growth, it will be suggested that you have monthly ultrasounds from at least 28 weeks, in addition to the routine ultrasounds offered earlier in the pregnancy. The estimated size of each baby will often be plotted on a graph so that it becomes more apparent if one or the other has started to slow down.

The other thing that may be monitored during pregnancy is the length of your cervix, usually measured by ultrasound. This is because twin pregnancies have a much higher chance of labour starting prematurely compared with single-baby pregnancies. Twin pregnancy is one of the most common risk factors for preterm birth. The reasons for this are more complicated than just having more weight on your cervix, and probably come down to a combination of mechanical and hormonal factors. If you are carrying twins and feel contractions earlier than your due date, you should definitely see your care provider.

Towards the end of the third trimester, you might also find that you are offered earlier-than-typical induction of labour, even before your due date or with no complications. This may be another example of doctors getting nervous and over-intervening, but the reason for this once again comes down to stillbirth prevention. In many ways, 37 weeks is more like full term for twins than 40 weeks. By nature, most twins come earlier than average. The rate of unexplained stillbirth for one or both twins is higher than with single-baby pregnancies and, like single pregnancies, the rate of this tragic occurrence starts to climb after the due date. A decision to avoid an induction as a twin pregnancy approaches or goes beyond 40 weeks gestation should prompt a little more caution and observation to make sure the babies are doing well, and the placentas are keeping up.

How to deliver: natural or caesarean?

Twin birth is amazing, but it also comes with a few extra challenges.

Over the last decade or so, there has been a lot of research on the safest way to deliver twins. Now that caesarean birth has become so common and relatively safe, the big question is whether all women with twins should be offered elective caesarean as a preferred choice for delivery.

The consensus seems to be that there are no statistically significant safety advantages for caesarean birth over natural birth when it comes to twins. Most obstetricians will leave the question to the woman's preference. After a discussion about what is involved during twin birth, women will generally be offered the choice of natural labour or elective caesarean birth as long as there are no other complicating factors that would make a vaginal birth more of a risk.

The one additional factor that most obstetricians would not feel comfortable about is if the first twin is presenting breech when labour starts. Many obstetricians are nervous about breech birth when it comes to one baby. When you add the issues unique to twin birth, and the rare possibility of the two babies' heads locking during birth, most obstetricians shy away. If the second twin is breech – no problem. Second twin breech birth is very common and most obstetricians would be comfortable with this, even if they don't typically offer breech birth for single-baby pregnancies.

If you decide to have an elective caesarean, don't feel pressured, as this is a very reasonable choice. If you do aim for a natural birth, the additional steps and potential complications are discussed below.

First stage

The first stage of labour is basically the same as with one baby, except that we need to keep an eye on two heartbeats. Sometimes, the extra stretch on the uterus can make the contractions a little bit more erratic, but conversely the extra weight on the cervix can help it to be softer and stretchier leading in to birth. Induction of labour (if needed) is essentially the same.

All pain-relief options are still available; however, you may find that your obstetrician advises you to have an epidural. Many hospitals or obstetricians will have a policy about recommending epidural anaesthetic routinely for twin pregnancies during labour. In principle, this should not be mandatory. The reason for suggesting an epidural is mainly for the second stage (pushing part) due to the increased possibility of needing quick intervention. In theory, an epidural should decrease delays if a sudden intervention is needed.

The counterargument is that an epidural may interfere with some of the natural processes in second stage, which could make an intervention more likely. This is purely speculative though. It is still suggested that having a pre-existing epidural is probably safer when you are birthing twins.

Second stage

The beginning of the second stage is also just like with a single baby – push until it comes out. To be certain that we are listening to the heartbeats of both babies, it is possible you may be advised to use a fetal scalp electrode to listen to the heartbeat of the lowest twin (which is usually the harder of the two to keep track of with an external heartbeat sensor).

After the first baby comes out is when all the action happens in a twin birth. For the woman, all the relief and excitement and exhaustion of a normal birth happens just like with a single baby, and she will likely be focused on meeting her new child. The umbilical cord will generally be cut for the first twin, but the delivery of that placenta will wait until the second baby is out, and the first baby's cord will just stay where it is in the vagina, with the clamped end outside.

The contractions will often back off quite a bit after the first twin, even if an oxytocin infusion was used. The second amniotic sac will still be intact, and with the extra space inside the womb, the second baby has a lot more room to get into position for the second birth. This is where the possibility of complications arises.

The first thing the obstetrician needs to check is which way the second baby is trying to come out. This may not be the same way that it was lined up prior to the birth of the first twin. Second twins often change from head first to bottom first once there is all that extra space from delivering twin one. There are two things we do not want to be coming first though – the umbilical cord, or an arm. A baby cannot fit through the pelvis sideways, and the umbilical cord should always come out after the baby. The obstetrician will generally use an ultrasound machine to confirm the position of the second baby. If the baby is not lined up either head or bottom first, they may then apply some pressure on the abdomen to turn the baby into a more favourable position.

Once the second baby is lined up, the contractions need to come back into action. It is common for the contractions to back off quite a bit once the first baby is out, and the uterus needs to realise that it still has work to do. If the contractions are taking a long time to kick back in, an oxytocin infusion may be started.

There is no 'safe' time interval between the birth of twins, so long as the heartrate of the second twin is in normal range. Up to half an hour is generally considered to be normal. In most cases, it is much shorter, often less than 15 minutes. When the contractions have started again and the second baby is lined up, the obstetrician may break the waters of the second sac to let baby come down.

There is a small chance of something untoward happening when the waters break for the second twin. In this situation, the obstetrician may need to get baby out urgently. This could mean a caesarean for the second twin even after the first has come out naturally, an instrumental birth if it is head down and it can't be pushed out quickly, or, rarely, doing an internal manoeuvre to bring the baby out by the feet. The possibility of this is generally why an elective epidural is discussed with women birthing twins.

Third stage

When the babies are out, the uterus needs to contract down a lot more, as it has been overstretched, and there is twice as much placenta to come out. Due to the added risk for blood loss during this part of the birth, it is also more likely that your obstetrician will recommend using an oxytocin infusion to help the uterus contract quicker after the placenta is out. This part of the labour is otherwise the same as third stage for a single baby.

WHEN THERE IS ONLY ONE PLACENTA (MCDA)

The difference when twins share one placenta compared with each having their own is that the babies share their blood. All babies in the womb continuously cycle their blood through the placenta. When twins share a placenta, their umbilical cords insert into the placenta separately, but the blood inside the placenta mixes.

Just like in the body, blood vessels in the placenta are of two different types – arteries and veins. Arteries are where blood is pumped in, at high pressure. Veins are where blood is drained out, at lower pressure. With monochorionic twins, the arteries and veins from one twin can join with those of the other twin inside the placenta. If the balance of these joins (or anastomoses) favours one twin, then it is possible for one twin to get more blood back from the placenta than it pumped in, at the expense of the other twin. This is called twin to twin transfusion syndrome.

This unique possibility makes it important to monitor monochorionic twins early in the pregnancy with ultrasound, in order to detect early signs of any imbalance. Later in the pregnancy, growth of monochorionic twins is also monitored by ultrasound, but often more frequently than with dichorionic twins. A difference in the size between monochorionic twins is more likely to indicate a problem with the placenta than it might in dichorionic twins.

During the birth

Vaginal birth is still an option with MCDA twins, with the same considerations as DCDA twins. It is commonly recommended to consider inducing labour or having a caesarean earlier again with MCDA twins compared with DCDA, because late pregnancy complications related to the placenta are thought to be more common.

Most obstetricians will be comfortable going to at least 37 weeks if all else is well. The labour and birth for MCDA twins is essentially managed in the way as DCDA twins.

WHEN THERE IS ONLY ONE AMNIOTIC SAC (MCMA)

This is the least common type of twin pregnancy. If your twins share an amniotic sac, you will need very close monitoring with an experienced obstetrician throughout the pregnancy. The additional unique complication for MCMA twins is the possibility of cord entanglement. Because the babies are swimming around together in the one pool, there is a possibility of them getting their oxygen lines in a tangle. This can happen during the pregnancy or during labour.

You would be hard-pressed to find an obstetrician who would recommend vaginal birth with MCMA twins. This type of twin pregnancy is thought to be safest delivered by elective caesarean. As fluid naturally shrinks at the end of pregnancy, cord accidents are more frequent, and the rate of stillbirth climbs dramatically for MCMA twins compared with other types of twin pregnancy. For this reason, it is often recommended to consider having the babies much earlier, even by 34 weeks.

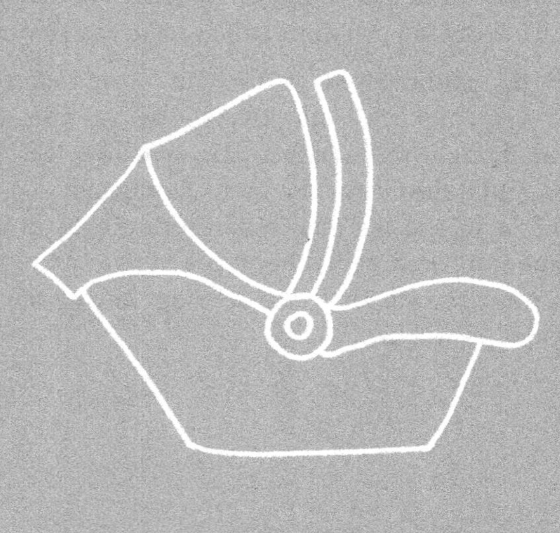

AFTER THE BIRTH

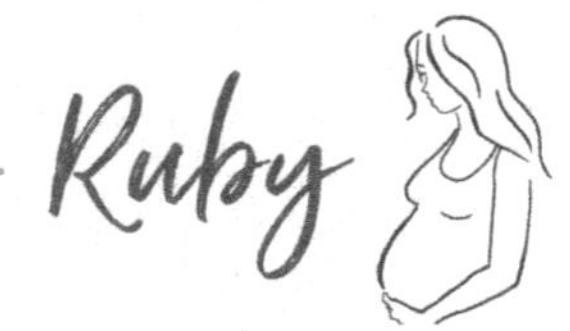

VAGINAL BIRTH RECOVERY

After a vaginal birth, you will most likely feel tender and sore. Whether or not you have stitches, give yourself the time to heal.

Tips for a comfortable recovery:

- Use ice packs – these will become your best friend for those first few days.
- Make sure you get plenty of rest. Lying down will take the pressure off your perineum, particularly if you have stitches.
- Take a 'sitz bath', a shallow bath for your hips and buttocks, which can ease pain and itching from your perineum. Salt baths can help, too.
- Avoid lifting anything heavier than your baby for the first few weeks.
- Be prepared for some bleeding. Wear loose, comfortable and dark-coloured clothing.
- Start pelvic floor exercises in the weeks following the birth.
- Nourish your body with healthy food, and stay hydrated particularly if you're breastfeeding.

What I'm really thinking:

The first hello

That first embrace is like no other feeling, a moment that I will never forget. Having a baby, from pregnancy to birth, is such a profound experience. Until I gave birth to my daughter, I didn't realise I could love someone so much. After the birth I was exhausted and overwhelmed, yet utterly and completely in love with and fascinated by my baby.

Newborn immunisations

Your newborn's first immunisations are usually given prior to leaving hospital. Your doctor or midwives will most likely discuss this with you when arriving at hospital or just after the birth.

Vitamin K – When your baby is born, they will have little to no vitamin K, as it does not cross the placenta from mother to baby during pregnancy. Vitamin K helps the blood to clot and therefore prevent excessive bleeding. It is given after birth to your baby to prevent haemorrhagic disease of the newborn (HDN) or serious bleeding, which can be fatal.

Hepatitis B – This is given to prevent the spread of disease from people who may be infected and come into contact with a newborn baby. It is safe and tolerated well by newborn babies, though minor side effects include redness and swelling at the site of the injection. It does not affect breastfeeding, and is given after birth, or within the first week.

Going to the toilet after giving birth

No one talks about it, and no one tells you, but going to the toilet for the first time after birth can be nerve-wracking. The midwife will ask many times whether you've passed wind (for a C-section) and had a bowel movement.

If you are worried or feel that you can't go to the toilet, ask for a stool softener to make the experience less daunting. A lot has happened 'down there'! Similarly, if you have had stitches, you may have a stinging, burning sensation or just feel uncomfortable when urinating at first. However, this will ease over the next few days or weeks as you begin to heal.

THE EARLY WEEKS

The first week can bring some challenges: taking baby home, getting to grips with feeding and the sleepless nights, and the all-important recovery of your own body. Finding your feet as a mother can take time, so don't place any pressure or expectations on yourself and reach out if you feel you need any help at all.

After you leave the hospital, you will receive a home visit from a midwife. There is no need to rush around making the house look tidy or getting the tea and biscuits out. The midwife visit is purely to support you and your baby. This is a great opportunity to ask for advice and discuss any concerns.

The midwife will not only check that baby is feeding well, but also how you are recovering and coping with bringing baby home. They may also ask you to fill out a questionnaire about your mental wellbeing to identify any signs of postnatal depression. They can also provide you with information as to where to go for weigh-ins and check-ups, support with breastfeeding or bottle-feeding, immunisation etc.

Postpartum sex

It is not uncommon to feel a little uneasy about resuming sex after birth. Most health professionals suggest waiting up to 6 weeks after giving birth before having sex, or until bleeding ceases. This is very much a personal choice and it might be earlier or later for you, depending on your birth experience and your recovery. Breastfeeding can cause vaginal dryness, so you may find using a lubricant is useful.

What I'm really thinking:

The 'baby blues'

Throughout my first pregnancy, I didn't think too much about how I would feel *after* the birth. I just wanted to get through the pregnancy and then focus on the birth experience. So the physical and mental toll of recovering from the birth, learning how to breastfeed and dealing with the 'baby blues' came as quite a surprise.

I had heard from other new mothers about the emotional low of day 3, but I brushed it aside, thinking I wouldn't experience it. Well, I was wrong. I did experience it, and for more than just one day. Day 3 came along and I was packing my bags to leave the hospital. Midwives were helping me get my baby ready, and I sat down and began to cry for no apparent reason. I couldn't pinpoint why I was crying or what triggered it, but I just sobbed. This occurred (usually around dinnertime) every night for about 4 or 5 days. Deep down, I felt loved and supported and so happy that my baby had made it into the world safely, but the profound change to my life overwhelmed me for a short while. It become much, much easier once my hormones started to settle and my baby and I got into a rhythm with breastfeeding and sleeping.

I would say to all new mothers: be kind to yourself. Ride the wave of emotions and ask for help along the way, whether it be from a family member, a friend or a health professional. Remember that your body is changing too. Take time to rest when baby is sleeping and don't put pressure on yourself to do anything other than live the experience.

BREASTFEEDING

Your breasts began making milk around week 16 of pregnancy. Some women notice milk leaking from their breasts during pregnancy, particularly in the later stages. This is not a cause for concern; your breasts are just getting ready for their important job ahead. After having your baby, the midwives will help you to navigate the ins and outs of breastfeeding. Your milk will come in anywhere from 48–96 hours after birth (day 2 to 4). Your breasts will feel swollen and full; they can also feel warm and tingly. These are all positive signs that your milk is coming in.

When your baby is first born, you will be advised to breastfeed on demand; as a guide, every 2–4 hours. Your baby may tend to feed less overnight and more frequently during the day. It can take time for babies to get to know night from day and get into a rhythm.

Breastfeeding is a skill that both you and your baby have to learn. Every woman will have a different experience with breastfeeding due to a few factors, including your baby, your breasts, your ability to produce milk and the latching of your baby onto the breast. It may take some time to get used to the sensations such as the let-down, tingling, latching and engorgement.

Don't feel disheartened if breastfeeding doesn't happen easily. The midwives are there to teach, support and guide you. Don't hesitate to reach out for advice from a specialist lactation consultant. Some babies have difficulties with latching on or colic; you may have an over-supply or a low supply of milk, or develop mastitis or thrush. These problems can affect any breastfeeding woman at any time and there are solutions. If you are experiencing any problems or just need to talk, there is plenty of support out there.

Some women are unable to breastfeed, which can be due to a variety of factors. If you don't produce quite enough milk, you have the option of combination feeding, when you give your baby breastmilk and then 'top up' with formula. When switching to combination feeding or bottle-feeding, some women can feel as though they have 'failed' at breastfeeding. It's important to remember that all women are different, just as all babies are different. There is no right or wrong way: whatever works best for you and your baby is perfect.

Tips for breastfeeding

- If you are experiencing any discomfort, place a cold flannel or cold gel pads onto your breast to help with any engorgement. Here's a DIY hack: my lovely midwife told me to place a couple of newborn nappies in the freezer until cold and use them instead – they really do the trick! It's also a good idea to alternate and drain each breast when feeding to give you some relief.
- Have a glass or bottle of water within reach, as you can get very thirsty while breastfeeding and it's easy to become dehydrated.
- Keep the breastfeeding helpline number in your phone – they provide support 7 days a week and are an incredible help.

What is colostrum?

The first milk your breasts make is called colostrum. You may have heard about 'liquid gold' and this is it. Oxytocin and prolactin, the hormones that are released after birth, are responsible for stimulating milk production and the supply to the nipple. Yellowish in colour and thick compared to milk, colostrum is what your baby will receive for a few days until your milk comes in. It is full of antibodies that will protect your little one and help them to build a strong immune system, and rich in vitamins and minerals.

What I'm really thinking:

Breastfeeding

When I first began breastfeeding, my breasts felt full, swollen and sore. I found that having a warm shower and allowing the milk to leak offered temporary relief . . . at least until my baby was awake or ready to feed. After a few days, once my baby started to get into a feeding routine (every 2 hours), my breasts became less tender and swollen. After the first 2 weeks, we finally got the hang of it. I felt more at ease holding him in the right positions, latching him onto the breast and then letting him feed until he released from the breast (or fell asleep).

BOTTLE-FEEDING

If you have chosen to bottle-feed, be sure to pack all the necessary equipment, including formula, bottles with newborn teats and a steriliser, in your hospital bag. Your breasts will still continue to make milk, so expect a bit of tenderness and engorgement after the birth. As your baby will not be stimulating the milk supply, this will slowly dwindle and you'll find that any discomfort will soon settle.

Tips for choosing formula:

- Check the tin to make sure the formula complies with Australian standards. Formula sold in the supermarket should meet these requirements.
- Always choose the right formula for the stage or age of your child. 'Stage 1' or 'Birth–12 months' formula contains the necessary nutrients for your newborn baby. 'Follow on' milks are for babies 12 months and older.
- Unless your baby has an allergy, purchasing formulas that are hypo-allergenic (HA) or soy-based may be unnecessary. Speak with your GP, child health nurse or midwife if you are unsure.
- Formula can vary from brand to brand when it comes to cost. 'Specialised' and 'organic' formulas tend to be more expensive.

The recommended temperature for prepared formula milk is 35–40°C. You can check this by either taking a sip (the milk should be just warm) or by dripping some of the milk onto your wrist. There are also kettles that boil and then reheat the water to 40°C.

Sterilising bottles

You will need to sterilise all your feeding equipment before every use, whether you are using bottles for formula or expressed breastmilk. You can use an electric or microwave steriliser, or simply sterilise in boiling water on the stovetop. To do this, place bottles, lids and teats in a saucepan and cover with water. Bring to the boil for 5 minutes, then leave to cool in the water before removing. Store in the fridge until use. Formula can leave a residue on the inside of the bottle, so it is a good idea to wash it in hot soapy water straight after use.

What I'm really thinking:

Bottle-feeding

At my antenatal classes the emphasis was on breastfeeding: it was all 'breast is best'. I think because of this I felt the pressure to breastfeed, even though I had issues with milk supply from the start. After 7 difficult months of trying to exclusively breastfeed, I decided to bottle-feed my daughter. At first, I felt disappointed and guilty. There can be a stigma around bottle-feeding, and sometimes I even felt embarrassed to give my baby a bottle in public. After a while, I realised that it was more important my baby was thriving than whether she was bottle-fed or breastfed.

There was so much to learn when it came to bottle-feeding. I had so many questions at first. How many bottles does my baby need over a day? How do I sterilise properly? Which formula is best? Which teats should I use? I asked friends and family what worked for them, and I tried and tested many formulas, using sample satchels where possible before having to purchase a whole tin of (expensive) formula. I found that the teats that worked best were the ones that mimicked the breast shape and size.

What I liked most about bottle-feeding was that my partner could be involved in feeding our daughter too. He would wake and give her a bottle at night, which was lovely bonding time for them. And if I was late home from work (or just needed a break), I didn't have to worry.

Danielle, mum of two

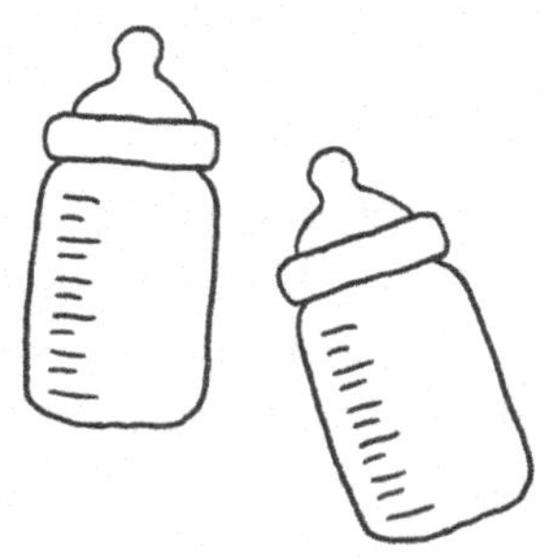

David

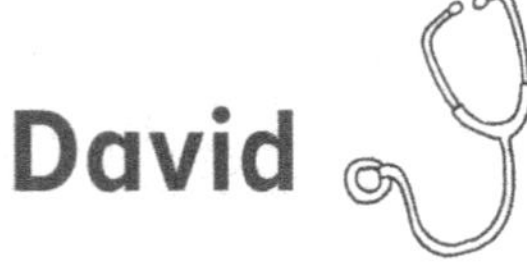

THE POSTNATAL CHECK-UP

The months after having a baby are filled with unexpected challenges and small miracles as you discover your child changing every day. Your body and emotions will also go through a lot of changes. Below are some important medical issues your obstetrician and midwife will be watching out for in the first days and weeks after birth. These are common issues that will be discussed in your postnatal check-up.

BLEEDING

This can initially be a little heavy in the first 24 hours, but then should settle down to period level, or less. The medical name for the bleeding that occurs after birth is lochia. It will usually have a different colour and odour to normal menstrual bleeding. Bleeding after birth will generally go on for a number of weeks, but usually is more or less gone by 6 weeks postnatal. It can be within normal limits to get a little bit of bleeding even up to 3 months from the birth.

If you notice increasing heaviness, fresher red bleeding, clots or an odour, this may not be normal and you should talk to a doctor. The main things the doctor will look for include whether there is any retained placental tissue in the uterus (using ultrasound), or whether there is a low-grade bacterial infection in the uterus.

How long it takes for your menstrual period to return varies between women and is influenced by breastfeeding patterns, as the hormone your brain produces to cause lactation also suppresses menstruation. For women who cannot breastfeed, or choose to formula-feed, it is common for periods to return quickly, often within 2 months of the birth. For women who exclusively breastfeed, periods commonly return 4 –6 months after birth. Breastfeeding and sleeping patterns for the baby have a strong influence. If you go for long stretches without breastfeeding (such as 8 hours, when baby starts sleeping through the night), it is more likely your hormones will start to reset, and you will start menstruating again. However, it is not unusual to get your period within a couple of months even if you are breastfeeding like a champ.

BREASTMILK

Breastmilk takes a few days to 'come in'. Once it is fully established, one of the most important factors to keep up supply is emptying the breasts regularly. This can be by feeding directly, or by using a breast pump if there are reasons baby is not attaching directly. The most common are when formula feeds are introduced, or when the baby starts sleeping through the night. In both cases, the reason is that there are longer gaps between feeds and the stimulus to keep milk flowing is reduced.

If milk supply becomes very difficult to maintain, despite trying physical stimulation, there are some remedies you can try. A herbal supplement called fenugreek can be very effective, and is available over-the-counter. Your doctor can also prescribe a medication called domperidone, which can also be effective in more problematic cases.

Rarely, women have medical conditions for which they are told not to breastfeed, and some women choose not to for personal reasons. There are natural methods for inhibiting milk production, but if this is a known plan, speak with your obstetrician in advance of the birth. There are medications available which, if given shortly afterwards, will inhibit milk production and save undue discomfort.

Below are some common barriers to breastfeeding, which can be addressed with a bit of advice from your doctor or midwife:

- Transiently blocked milk ducts causing pain.
- Nipple ulcers and cracks.
- Flat or indrawn nipples.
- Tongue-tie, small mouth or receded jawline (baby issues).

Most of these can be helped with some advice about technique. Sometimes a nipple shield may help. If there is a baby issue, review with a GP or paediatrician may also be helpful.

If one breast becomes red, painful and hot, you could have mastitis, which is an infection in the milk ducts. Ask a doctor or midwife to check, because antibiotics may be necessary. We recommend continuing to feed baby from that breast, even if there are signs of infection, as the bacteria involved will not harm baby's stomach, and emptying the breast regularly is very important for healing.

YOUR BLADDER

The most important thing about your bladder is to empty it regularly after the birth. A baby just pushed its way under your pubic bone and your urethra was squished in the process. There can be a significant amount of swelling in the skin of the vagina around the opening here as well. If there were tears that went upwards, odds are they will be within a few centimetres of the urethra, too. The combination of these things can make the prospect of doing a wee a little scary or a little difficult. If you had an epidural anaesthetic, this will also make your bladder a bit lazy as the nerves to your bladder take longer than the nerves to your legs to start working again.

Every now and then, we see women who have trouble emptying the bladder after having a baby and this can cause the bladder muscle to become overstretched. In this case, it may need a few days to get back in shape. This could mean a catheter is required to keep the bladder empty while the muscles tone up, and any swelling decreases. On the flipside, it is quite common to have a little bit of bladder weakness initially after giving birth. Don't be too alarmed if you have the occasional accident with a laugh, sneeze or cough, particularly if it is only in the first few days or weeks after baby. Things take time to tone up.

Occasionally, bladder weakness can persist beyond the postnatal period. Weakness from pressure on the bladder is called urinary stress incontinence. If this is a persistent problem, you definitely need to work on pelvic floor exercises. A physiotherapist with an interest in pelvic floor training can be very informative. For severe cases, there are surgeries that can correct this, but usually surgery will only be recommended after you have finished having babies.

YOUR STITCHES (AND PELVIC FLOOR)

Only dissolvable stitches should be used in the vagina and pelvic floor after birth. This means that there is nothing that needs to be removed. In most cases, I tell women to try to forget about the stitches they have had (if they are able to) since the odds are that they are healing up perfectly fine. There is nothing special you have to do down there, just keep things generally clean and dry. Infections in perineal stitches are very uncommon. Don't use antiseptics or harsh soaps, as these may irritate the area, and antibacterial agents may encourage resistant infections. If things feel more swollen or sore over time, it is possible something is not right, so speak up. If you feel that things have come apart, or the skin edges are not sitting together properly, see your doctor or midwife. Even if there is an area where the skin has separated, unless things are really bad, often it is better to let things heal before having a repeat procedure to repair the area.

Many women ask when they can start doing their pelvic floor exercises after birth. There is no right answer, and if things feel comfortable, you can start doing them whenever you like. It is probably wise to avoid putting the stitches to the test for the first couple of weeks.

CONTRACEPTION AND/OR PLANNING FOR NEXT TIME

There is no right or wrong time to start having sex again, as long you feel comfortable, but a lot of women leave it a few weeks before trying. As mentioned, it can be quite variable in how long it takes for your period to return after having a baby, and this is significantly impacted by breastfeeding patterns. It is true that breastfeeding offers some natural contraception by suppressing the menstrual period; however, a period happens 2 weeks *after* you ovulate. This means that if you wait for your period to come back before worrying about contraception, you ovulated for the first time 2 weeks before that period. Women can (and do) get pregnant again after a baby without ever getting a period.

Barrier methods (e.g. condoms) are fine to use when breastfeeding. If you use 'natural' methods to time ovulation and your fertile window, be aware that your hormones might not be so predictable for a while until your menstrual cycle kicks back in.

If you want something on prescription for contraception and you are still breastfeeding, the answer is progesterone-only contraception. The difference between these types and the typical combined contraceptive pill is the omission of oestrogen. This is because oestrogen can have a negative effect on your breastmilk supply. Not having oestrogen in the pill means that you don't get a scheduled period, and there are no sugar tablet breaks, like in a typical contraceptive pill.

There are four ways that progesterone contraception can be given:

- A daily tablet, often called the mini-pill.
- An injection every 3 months.
- An implant in your arm, which can last for up to 3 years.
- A device inserted into the uterus (an IUD), which is put in with a minor procedure a bit like a longer pap smear.

The first three types can be started as soon as you like after birth. The IUD is recommended from after 6 weeks, when the uterus is back to normal size. The oral progesterone pill is also a little more prone to failure than a normal contraceptive pill, and it is very important to take it at the same time every day, and not to rely on it if you have other things impacting metabolism, such as strong antibiotics. The other three are generally more reliable than the oral pill for contraception.

How soon can I go again?

This depends on the circumstances of your birth, and how you feel about adding another pregnancy to the mix. In general, if your body lets you fall pregnant again, it is ready. It is definitely something to talk with your obstetrician about, especially if there were any complications around your birth, such as bad tears, infection or a complicated caesarean. There are some potential physical advantages to waiting a little longer between babies, especially when it comes to abdominal muscle and pelvic-floor recovery.

MEDICAL CONDITIONS

As mentioned earlier, there are some surprise conditions that can pop up during pregnancy. Some of these can have implications on your health, even after the baby is out, and will require a few check-ups to make sure things are back to normal. The most common examples are high blood pressure (or preeclampsia) and gestational diabetes. There is a small chance that these conditions will persist after the baby is born, though in most cases, things go back to normal pretty soon. Getting these conditions during pregnancy may also be a warning sign that you are at risk of developing them as chronic medical conditions later in life. For example, women who have gestational diabetes have a 50 per cent chance of lifestyle-related type 2 diabetes.

Having a medical condition arise during your pregnancy may also have some implications on future pregnancies. In some cases, there are things that might be done differently or earlier in a new pregnancy to give the best chance of avoiding the condition coming back or reducing its severity. There are also a number of medical conditions that women may have prior to getting pregnant, which are significantly altered by pregnancy. Examples include autoimmune conditions, which often have a tendency to improve during pregnancy but may flare up significantly in the postnatal period. Certain long-term medications may need to have dose adjustments during pregnancy, and then again after the birth. A common example of this is thyroid hormone replacement.

MOOD AND COPING

Most women experience emotional highs and lows during the postnatal period. If minor mood changes, moments of helplessness and feelings of frustration are happening from time to time, know this is very common and doesn't mean you are not an excellent mother. It is important to let people know how you are feeling about your experiences, though, and your doctor or midwife is a good first point of contact. It is definitely important to involve family and loved ones in your emotional experiences. A professional support person will be able to see things from a different perspective than partners, parents and friends.

There are a few common times when women may be challenged emotionally in the postnatal period. Days 3 to 4 after the birth are a common low point (often called the postnatal or 'baby blues') and I imagine it has at least a little to do with the hormonal changes that are going on as the breastmilk comes in. It is not uncommon to feel teary and upset, and to not even know why you might be feeling this way. It is important for partners (and doctors) to not take these emotions personally, but to be available and open for support as needed. It is becoming increasingly common for women to be encouraged to go home very early after birth (even within the first day), so often this low point can be missed during a hospital stay. Most birth services will offer further support by contact with midwives and doctors by phone or home visits after leaving hospital to make sure things aren't becoming overwhelming after you take baby home.

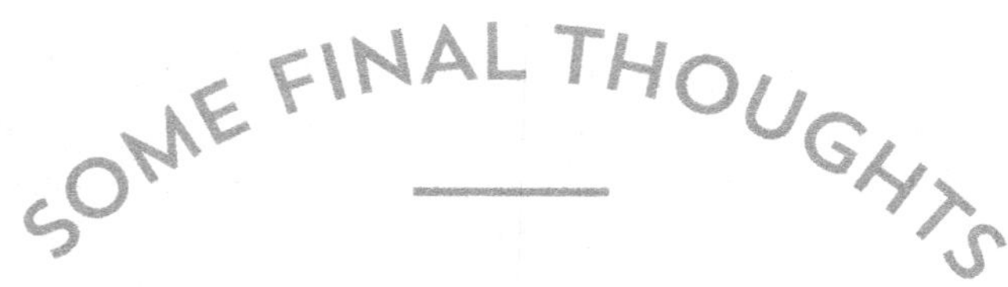

David

Birth is an experience that many women may have only once, or a few times in their life. By all means – plan for this experience, cherish it and make it your own. Reading books, like this one, talking with friends and listening to the experiences of others are all great ways to be prepared.

I have one of the best jobs in the world, because I have the opportunity to vicariously experience birth almost every day. I have seen some amazing things, and some tragic things, but I have not seen it all. I continue to be surprised and educated by my patients each day. Most of what I know about pregnancy and birth has not come from research papers and textbooks, but from watching and listening to the women who are doing it.

Make use of the experience of your doctors and midwives to shape your birth. Listen to their advice, but please feel free to question it. The ideally supported birth is a team effort, with you at the centre, and those around you should always have the best interests of you and your baby in mind.

I hope that the information in this book is useful, but I know that not everything applies to all women and each pregnancy.

There is no substitute for the real thing. If you haven't already, find a doctor or a midwife who can find out about your story and help you navigate your own path.

Safe travels and best wishes,

David

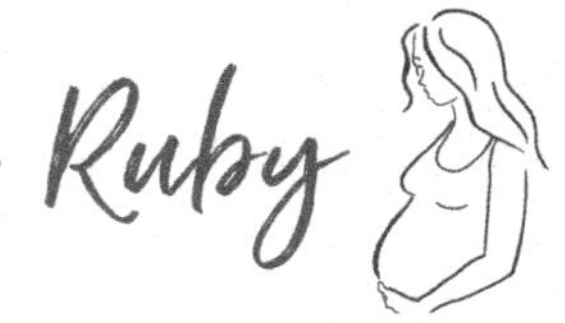

I hope that by reading this book you feel more confident, calm and reassured about your pregnancy, birth and the first week of your little one's life. I hope that the countless questions I had in both my pregnancies are answered here for you, so that you feel equipped to make decisions and feel more at ease.

I also hope you will place importance on your mental health and wellbeing throughout your pregnancy. Relish the joyful moments – the first fluttery kicks, the first time you hear the heartbeat or see your baby on ultrasound – and remember to let go of unrealistic expectations.

Don't underestimate your strength; believe in your ability to grow and birth your baby; and trust your instincts. Pass this book on to your partner or support person to read so they too can understand how to better support you through your pregnancy journey.

Those first moments and weeks when your baby enters the world can be surreal. Allow your body to rest and recover. Never be afraid to ask for help. Let time pass you by, as you enjoy those moments of watching your baby simply breathe and sleep. Notice the tiny fingers and toes, that perfectly round button nose; bask in the beauty of the fact that you and your partner have created this little person.

A nurse once told me that we must take care of ourselves before we can take care of our baby and I wholeheartedly believe in this. As new mothers, we often forget about our own needs. Even with the demands of caring for our baby, we must take the time for ourselves when we can.

And when you look back on these past 9 months, the difficult days of soreness and sickness will soon fade as you focus on the life-changing and monumental experience of raising your beautiful little baby.

With love, Ruby

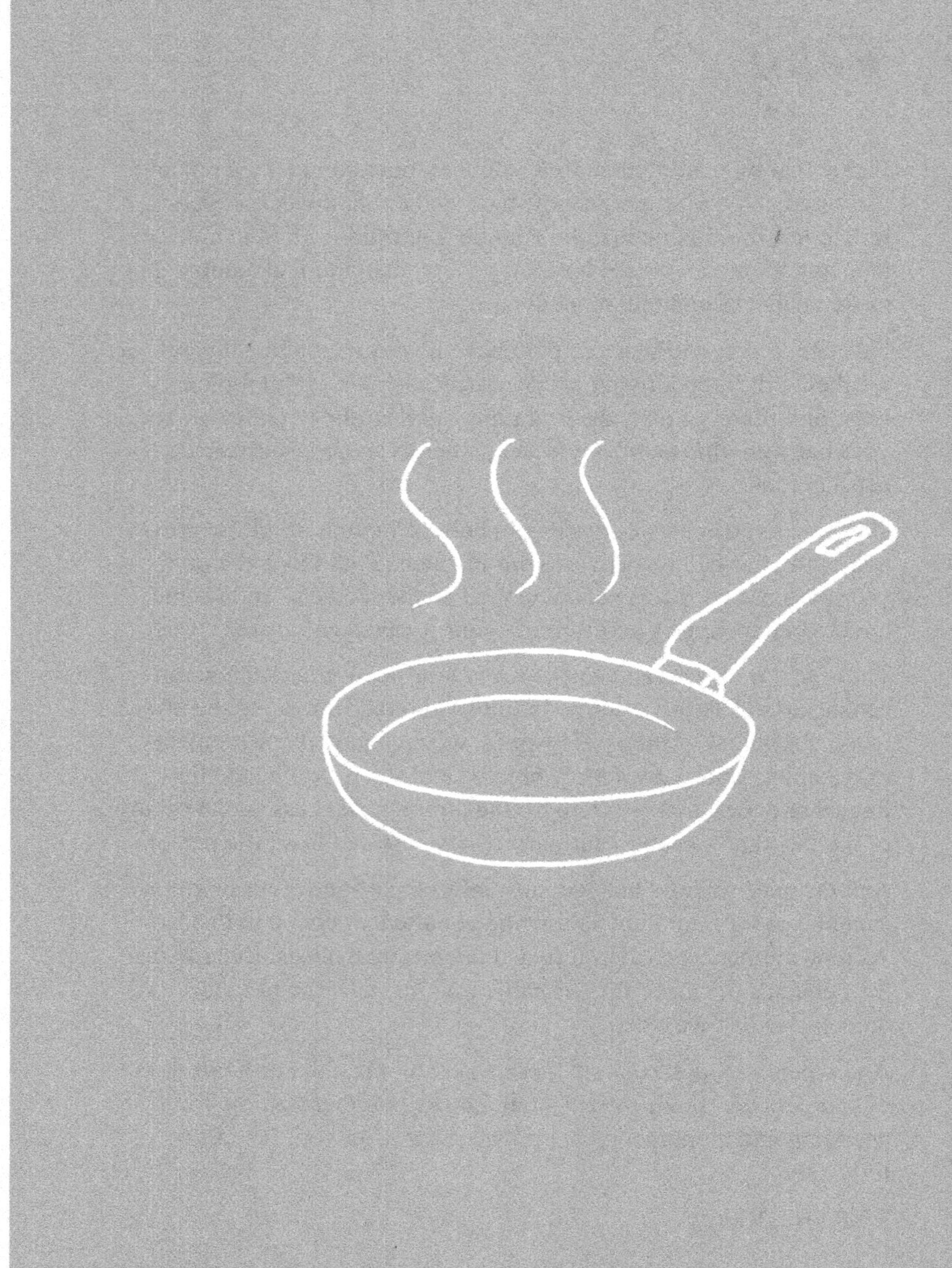

RECIPES

BREAKFAST

Banana protein smoothie

¾ cup milk of your choice
1 banana
2 tablespoons Greek yoghurt
2 teaspoons chia seeds
1 tablespoon shredded coconut
1 tablespoon LSA or almond meal

Place all the ingredients in a blender and whizz to combine.

Green smoothie

½ cup milk of your choice
½ cup coconut water
1 apple, chopped
½ banana
½ cucumber
1 teaspoon chia seeds
mint leaves, to taste

Place all the ingredients in a blender and whizz to combine.

Berry avo smoothie

½ cup milk of your choice
½ cup coconut water
½ cup blueberries
½ cup strawberries, hulled
¼ avocado
handful of baby spinach leaves

Place all the ingredients in a blender and whizz to combine.

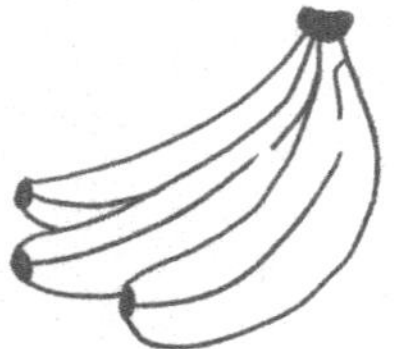

Overnight oats

½ cup milk of your choice
½ cup rolled oats
¼ cup natural yoghurt
¼ cup fruit, nuts and/or seeds

Place the milk, oats and yoghurt in a large glass jar. Stir to combine. Add your choice of fruit, nuts and/or seeds – try raspberries, slivered almonds and chia seeds, or strawberries, chopped pecans and sunflower seeds (or try the combination below). Place in the fridge overnight, ready to eat in the morning.

Blueberry, hazelnut & chia overnight oats

½ cup milk of your choice
½ cup rolled oats
¼ cup hazelnuts, chopped
1 tablespoon chia seeds
1 teaspoon ground cinnamon
¼ cup blueberries

Place the milk, oats, hazelnuts and chia seeds in a large glass jar. Stir to combine, and add the cinnamon. Place in the fridge overnight. Add the blueberries before serving.

Vanilla porridge with stewed fruit

1 cup quick oats
½ cup milk of your choice
1 teaspoon vanilla extract
2 tablespoons almond meal
1 tablespoon Greek yoghurt

Stewed fruit
2 apples, 2 pears or 4 rhubarb stems, chopped

For the stewed fruit, place your choice of fruit in a saucepan with ¼ cup water. Simmer over medium heat until the fruit has softened, then leave to cool. Transfer to a glass container and store in the fridge for up to 3 days.

Place the oats in a saucepan with the milk and ¼ cup water. Cook over low heat for 4 minutes, then stir in the vanilla and almond meal.

Transfer the porridge to a serving bowl and top with yoghurt and stewed fruit.

Quick veggie eggs

2 free-range eggs
¼ cup milk
sea salt and black pepper
2 tablespoons olive oil
1 large flat mushroom, sliced
½ cup baby spinach leaves
100 g feta

Whisk the eggs in a bowl with the milk. Season with salt and pepper. Heat the oil in a frying pan over medium–high heat. Add the mushroom and cook for 1–2 minutes, then add the spinach and cook for a further minute or until wilted.

Pour in the egg mixture and cook for 4 minutes, lightly stirring every minute or so, then add the feta. Cook until the eggs are light and fluffy and no liquid remains. Slide the eggs from the pan and serve immediately.

Serves 2

Avocado on sourdough

1 tablespoon olive oil
5 cherry tomatoes, halved
sea salt and black pepper
½ avocado, mashed
1–2 slices sourdough toast
freshly squeezed lemon, to taste

Heat the oil in a frying pan over medium–high heat and add the tomatoes. Season with salt and pepper and saute until softened.

Spread the mashed avocado onto the toasted sourdough.

Squeeze over the lemon juice and enjoy.

Quinoa breakfast bowl

1 free-range egg
½ cup quinoa
½ avocado, sliced
4 cherry tomatoes, halved
handful of baby spinach leaves
2 tablespoons goat's cheese
dill fronds, to serve
sesame seeds, to serve
freshly squeezed lemon, to taste

Place the egg in a saucepan with 3 cups cold water and bring to the boil. Boil for 6–8 minutes, then turn off the heat and leave for up to 10 minutes to make sure the egg is cooked through and the yolk is no longer runny.

Meanwhile, rinse the quinoa in a colander, then place in a saucepan with 1 cup water and a pinch of salt. Cook over medium heat for 10 minutes or until the quinoa has absorbed the water.

Slice the hard-boiled egg and place in a bowl with the avocado, tomato, spinach, goat's cheese and quinoa. Sprinkle with dill and sesame seeds. Squeeze over lemon to taste.

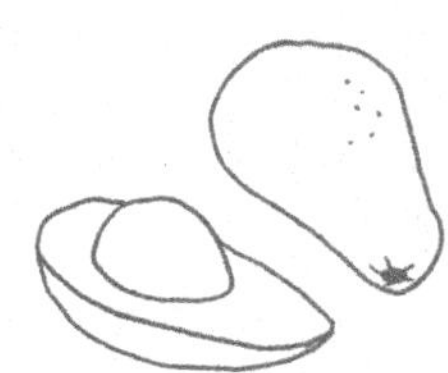

SNACKS

Ginger & lemon cordial

5 cm knob ginger, peeled
1 teaspoon honey
juice of 2 lemons

Finely chop the ginger and place in a saucepan with 1 litre water. Bring to the boil over high heat, then reduce the heat to low and simmer for 5 minutes.

Strain the liquid into a jug, discarding the ginger. Stir through the honey, then set aside to cool.

Once the cordial is cool, add the lemon juice. Store in the fridge.

This refreshing drink is especially good for first-trimester nausea.

Good-for-you banana bread

3 overripe bananas
3 free-range eggs
2 tablespoons honey
45 ml olive or macadamia oil
1 teaspoon vanilla extract
1 cup almond meal
¼ cup shredded coconut

Preheat the oven to 180°C (160°C fan-forced) and line a loaf tin with baking paper.

Mash the bananas in a large bowl and add the eggs, honey, oil and vanilla. Mix well. Fold the almond meal into the mixture, then add the coconut and stir well.

Transfer the mixture to the prepared tin.

Bake for 25–30 minutes or until golden on top and cooked through. Remove from the oven and allow to sit for 5–10 minutes before serving.

Store in a sealed container in the fridge and eat within 5 days.

Chocolate bliss balls

6 medjool dates, pitted and chopped
1 teaspoon raw cacao powder
¼ cup almond meal
¼ cup hazelnuts (or hazelnut meal)
1 teaspoon hot water
¼ cup shredded coconut

Place the dates, cacao, almond meal, hazelnuts and hot water in a high-speed blender and blitz to combine (about 2–3 minutes). Place the coconut in a bowl. Roll the cacao mixture into small balls (you should have about 10), then coat with the coconut, placing them on a plate as you go. Chill for 4–6 hours before eating. Store in the fridge.

Strawberry bliss balls

6 medjool dates, pitted and chopped
5 strawberries, hulled
¼ cup rolled oats
¼ cup almond meal
½ cup shredded coconut

Place the dates, strawberries, oats and almond meal in a high-speed blender and blitz to combine (about 2–3 minutes). Place the coconut in a bowl. Roll the strawberry mixture into small balls (you should have about 10), then coat with the coconut, placing them on a plate as you go. Chill for 4–6 hours before eating. Keep in the fridge.

Apple & nut butter slices

1 apple, thinly sliced
2 tablespoons nut butter of your choice

Simply spread your nut butter over the sliced apple. A perfect go-to snack when you are feeling peckish.

Sweet potato & quinoa bites

1 sweet potato, peeled and chopped
1 cup quinoa
1 tablespoon olive oil
½ onion, finely chopped
½ garlic clove, finely diced
½ cup grated cheddar cheese

Preheat the oven to 200°C (180°C fan-forced) and grease a baking tray.

Bring a saucepan of water to the boil. Add the sweet potato, then reduce the heat to medium and cook for 10–15 minutes until the potato is soft. Drain, then transfer to a large bowl and mash until smooth.

Meanwhile, rinse the quinoa in a colander, then place in a saucepan with 2 cups water and a pinch of salt. Cook over medium heat for 10–15 minutes or until the quinoa has absorbed all the water. Add the quinoa to the sweet potato and combine well.

Heat the oil in a frying pan over medium–high heat and saute the garlic and onion for 1–2 minutes until softened. Add to the quinoa mixture along with the cheese and combine.

Place tablespoons of the mixture on the prepared tray to make about 12 bite-sized balls. Bake for 25–30 minutes or until golden.

Store in the fridge in a sealed container.

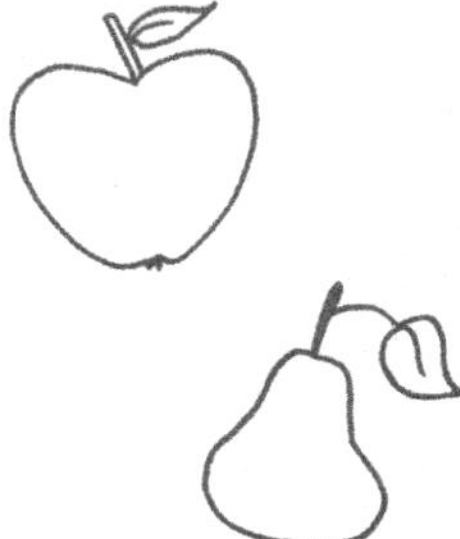

Date, nut & seed bars

½ cup raw cashews
¼ cup almond meal
½ cup hazelnuts
¼ cup sunflower seeds
5 medjool dates, pitted and chopped
½ cup nut butter
¼ cup shredded coconut

Place the cashews, almond meal, hazelnuts and sunflower seeds in a food processor and combine until the nuts are very finely chopped. Add the dates, nut butter and 2 tablespoons water and blitz to a dough-like consistency. Add the coconut and pulse until just combined.

Line a baking tray with baking paper. Transfer the dough to the prepared tray and use a fork to press down evenly. Place in the fridge overnight.

Transfer to a chopping board and slice into 8–10 bars. Store in a sealed container in the fridge.

Seasonal fruit salad & yoghurt

½ apple, chopped
(or whatever is in season)
½ cup berries
(or whatever is in season)
½ banana, chopped
Greek yoghurt or coconut yoghurt, to serve
crushed Trail mix (see below), to serve

Gently combine the fruit and store in a sealed container in the fridge. Serve with yoghurt and trail mix.

Trail mix

handful each of goji berries, coconut flakes, raw almonds, raw cashews and raw peanuts

Combine all the ingredients and store in a glass jar or container in the fridge.

LUNCH

French salad

1 cup canned green lentils, drained and rinsed
1 tomato, diced
¼ red onion, diced
50 g feta, crumbled
juice of ½ lemon
olive oil, for drizzling

Toss the lentils, tomato and onion together in a bowl. Add the feta and lemon juice. Drizzle with olive oil to taste. This simple salad can be eaten by itself or served on a slice of sourdough or crispbread.

Mediterranean lunch bowl

½ cup quinoa
½ cup canned chickpeas, drained and rinsed
½ cucumber, sliced
½ red capsicum, seeded and sliced
¼ red onion, finely sliced
6 cherry tomatoes, halved
juice of ¼ lemon
1 teaspoon Dijon mustard
1 tablespoon olive oil
sea salt and black pepper
50 g feta cheese, crumbled

Rinse the quinoa in a colander, then place in a saucepan with 1 cup water and a pinch of salt. Cook over medium heat for 10–15 minutes or until the quinoa has absorbed the water.

Place the quinoa, chickpeas, cucumber, capsicum, onion and tomatoes in a bowl.

Combine the lemon, mustard, olive oil, salt and pepper.

Drizzle the dressing over the salad and top with crumbled feta.

Pumpkin & ginger soup

1 tablespoon olive oil
2 cloves garlic, crushed
1 cm knob ginger, peeled and grated
1 onion, diced
1 small pumpkin, cubed
1 sweet potato, cubed
1 large potato, cubed
1 carrot, cubed
1 zucchini, cubed
2 cups vegetable stock
½ teaspoon ground cumin

Heat the olive oil in a saucepan over medium–high heat and saute the garlic, ginger and onion for 1–2 minutes until softened. Add the pumpkin, sweet potato, potato, carrot and zucchini. Cook for 2 minutes to brown, then add the vegetable stock and 1 litre water. Reduce the heat and simmer for 20 minutes until the vegetables become tender, then add the cumin. Leave to cool a little, then transfer to a blender and blend until smooth. Keep leftovers in the fridge for up to 3 days.

Six easy crispbread toppings

Avocado, tomato & cottage cheese

Top 2 crispbreads with ½ mashed avocado, 1 sliced tomato and 2 heaped tablespoons cottage cheese. Season with salt and pepper to taste.

Tuna, cheddar & tomato

Top 2 crispbreads with sliced cheddar cheese, 1 small can of tuna in oil or spring water and 1 sliced tomato.

Bruschetta-style

Top 2 crispbreads with 1 sliced tomato, ¼ sliced red onion and ½ clove crushed garlic. Drizzle with balsamic vinegar and garnish with basil.

Cucumber, avocado & feta cheese

Top 2 crispbreads with ½ mashed avocado, ¼ sliced cucumber and ¼ cup feta.

Hard-boiled egg, hummus & tomato

Top 2 crispbreads with a sliced hard-boiled egg, ¼ cup hummus and 1 sliced tomato.

Rocket, avo, tuna & spring onion

Top 2 crispbreads with ¼ mashed avocado, 1 small can of tuna, a handful of rocket and a sprinkling of sliced spring onion.

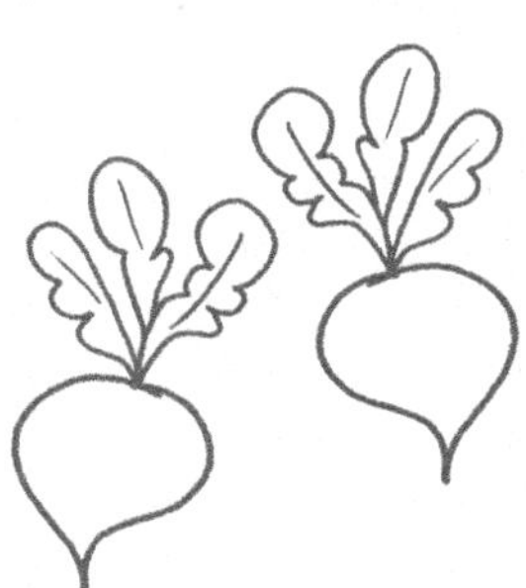

Nicoise salad

2 baby potatoes, boiled
10 green beans
1 hard-boiled free-range egg (page 259)
1 cup chopped lettuce
½ red onion, sliced
handful of cherry tomatoes
1 small can of tuna, drained
½ teaspoon Dijon mustard
juice of ½ lemon
1 tablespoon olive oil
sea salt and black pepper

Bring a saucepan of water to the boil and add the potatoes. Boil for up to 10 minutes or until you can easily pierce them with a fork, then drain.

Place the beans in a bowl, cover with boiling water and leave for 5 minutes, then drain and refresh under cold water.

Peel and slice the hard-boiled egg.

Arrange the lettuce, onion and tomatoes in a bowl. Add the egg, potatoes, beans and tuna.

Combine the mustard, lemon juice, oil, salt and pepper and drizzle over the salad before serving.

Wholesome tuna salad sandwich

¼ avocado, sliced
2 slices good wholemeal bread
¼ cup grated carrot
¼ cucumber, sliced
1 tomato, sliced
¼ zucchini, grated
1 slice beetroot
1 small can of tuna, drained
2 mint leaves, finely chopped
2 lettuce leaves

Place the avocado over one slice of bread and top with carrot, cucumber, tomato, zucchini and beetroot.

Add the tuna and top with mint leaves and lettuce. Add the remaining slice of bread and enjoy.

DINNER

Ginger soy fish & rice

1 cup rice (white, basmati or brown)
1 bunch bok choy
handful of green beans
1 bunch broccolini
handful of snow peas
200 g white fish (snapper or kingfish), cut into 3 cm pieces
1 teaspoon white wine vinegar
2 tablespoons soy sauce
2 teaspoons peanut oil
2 cm knob ginger, grated
2 spring onions, finely chopped
2 tablespoons chopped coriander
lime wedges, to serve

Place the rice in a saucepan with 2 cups of water and bring to the boil. Reduce the heat and simmer for 15 minutes until the water has been absorbed, then set aside and keep warm.

Steam the bok choy, beans and broccolini for 3–4 minutes over a saucepan of simmering water, then add the snow peas and steam for 1 minute.

Place the vinegar and ¼ cup water in a saucepan over medium heat and add the fish. Poach for 3–5 minutes or until cooked through.

Combine the soy sauce and peanut oil in a small bowl.

Divide the rice between two plates and add the fish. Top with the steamed vegetables, ginger, spring onion and coriander. Dress with the soy sauce and peanut oil. Squeeze lime over the top to serve.

Serves 2

Vegetarian soft tacos

1 tablespoon olive oil
1 clove garlic, crushed
1 red onion, chopped
2 small mushrooms, sliced
1 sweet potato, chopped
400 g can diced tomatoes
400 g can black beans or kidney beans
1 teaspoon paprika
½ teaspoon ground cumin
½ teaspoon dried oregano
sea salt and black pepper
¼ teaspoon chilli powder (optional)
2 soft corn tortilla wraps
1 cup grated cheese
1 avocado, mashed
Greek yoghurt and lime wedges, to serve

Heat the olive oil in a saucepan over high heat. Add the garlic and onion and saute for 1–2 minutes, then add the mushroom and fry for another 2 minutes. Add the sweet potato and cook for a further 1–2 minutes.

Add the tomatoes, beans and ¼ cup water, then reduce the heat to low. Simmer for 15 minutes, until the sweet potato is tender. Stir through the paprika, cumin, oregano and chilli, if using, and simmer for a few minutes more.

Serve the bean mixture on soft corn tortillas topped with mashed avocado, cheese and yoghurt, and lime wedges for squeezing over. Store any leftover bean mixture in the fridge for up to 3 days.

Serves 2

Chicken & vegetable soup

1.25 litres chicken stock or broth
400 g boneless, skinless chicken thighs
1 tablespoon olive oil
2 cloves garlic, crushed
1 onion, diced
2 carrots, diced
2 stalks celery, diced
1 zucchini, cubed
1 head broccoli, chopped into florets
1 bay leaf
2 teaspoons Worcestershire sauce
grated parmesan, to serve

Heat 1 cup stock in a saucepan over high heat and add the chicken. Poach for 2 minutes, then remove the chicken and set aside in a bowl in the fridge.

Heat the olive oil in a large saucepan over medium heat. Fry the garlic and onion for 1–2 minutes, then add the carrot, celery, broccoli, zucchini and bay leaf. Pour in the remaining stock, cover and simmer for 15 minutes. Add the Worcestershire sauce.

Shred the chicken thighs and add to the pan. Reduce the heat to low and cook for a further 5–10 minutes.

Serve the soup with grated parmesan.

Serves 2

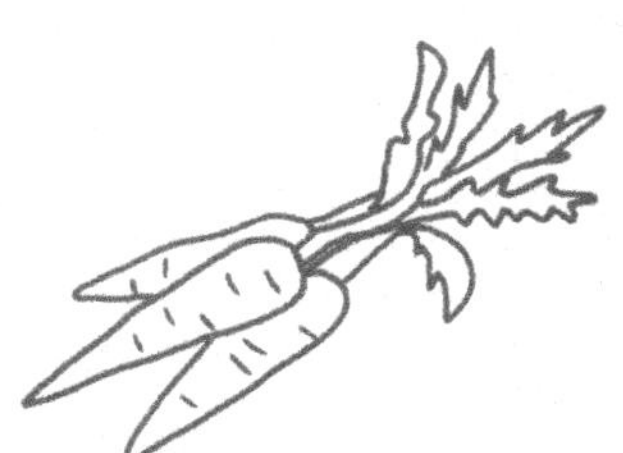

Asian chicken with slaw

1 tablespoon olive oil
1 clove garlic, chopped
1 cm knob ginger, chopped
¼ cup tamari or soy sauce
lemon juice, to taste
sea salt and black pepper
200 g chicken breast

Slaw

½ cup finely sliced green cabbage
¼ cup finely sliced red cabbage
½ cup chopped green capsicum
1 carrot, finely chopped
handful of raw almonds
1 cup rocket
¼ cup crunchy Asian-style noodles (optional)
¼ cup chopped spring onion
2 teaspoons tamari or soy sauce
1 teaspoon white vinegar
1 teaspoon olive oil

Preheat the oven to 200°C (180°C fan-forced).

Combine the oil, garlic, ginger, tamari, lemon juice, salt and pepper in a small bowl. Place the chicken on a baking tray and pour over the tamari mixture. Bake for 15 minutes or until the chicken is cooked through.

Place all the slaw ingredients in a bowl. Toss to combine and coat with the dressing.

Serve the chicken with the slaw.

Serves 2

Teriyaki salmon parcels

2 x 150 g salmon fillets
1 cup broccoli florets
2 mushrooms, thinly sliced
1 zucchini, thinly sliced
10–15 green beans
1 cup brown rice

Teriyaki sauce

¼ cup soy sauce or tamari
1 teaspoon Dijon mustard
1 clove garlic, finely chopped
1 teaspoon honey
1 tablespoon olive oil

Preheat the oven to 220°C (200°C fan-forced).

Cut two pieces of baking paper and place a salmon fillet in the centre of each. Top with the broccoli, mushrooms and zucchini.

Combine the teriyaki sauce ingredients in a small bowl and drizzle over the top.

Fold over both sides of the baking paper. Twist both ends to seal. Carefully transfer to a baking tray and bake for 20 minutes or until cooked through.

Meanwhile, place the rice and 2 cups of water in a saucepan and bring to the boil. Reduce the heat and cook for 15 minutes until the water is absorbed, then leave to rest with the lid on.

Place the beans in a heatproof bowl and cover with boiling water. Leave for 3 minutes, then drain and refresh.

Serve the fish parcels with the brown rice and green beans on the side.

Serves 2

Chicken & sweet potato curry

400 g boneless, skinless chicken thighs, cut into 3 cm pieces
2 tablespoons curry powder
1 tablespoon olive oil
1 red onion, chopped
4 cm knob ginger, grated
1 clove garlic, crushed
400 ml chicken stock
1 lemongrass stalk
2 tablespoons fish sauce
1 sweet potato, chopped
1 cup brown rice
150 ml coconut milk
coriander leaves and lemon wedges, to serve

Place the chicken in a shallow bowl and toss with the curry powder until coated.

Heat the olive oil in a saucepan over medium–high heat. Fry the onion, ginger and garlic until the onion is translucent. Add the chicken and fry until lightly browned. Pour in the stock and add the lemongrass, fish sauce and sweet potato. Reduce the heat to low and simmer for 15 minutes or until the sweet potato is tender. Stir in the coconut milk and warm through.

Meanwhile, place the rice and 2 cups of water in a saucepan and bring to the boil. Reduce the heat and cook for 15 minutes until the water is absorbed, then leave to rest with the lid on.

Garnish the curry with coriander and serve with rice and lemon wedges.

Serves 2

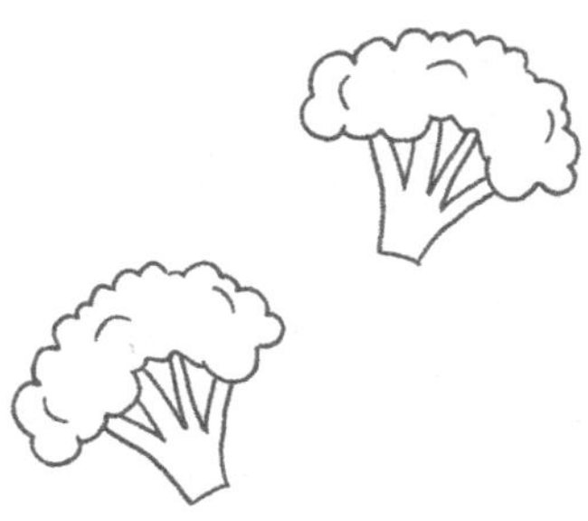

Lamb cutlets with mash & greens

4 lamb cutlets
1 clove garlic, sliced
2 teaspoons rosemary leaves
2 tablespoons olive oil
2 potatoes, cubed
3 tablespoons milk
1 teaspoon butter
1 bunch of broccolini

Preheat the oven to 200°C (180°C fan-forced).

Place the lamb cutlets on a baking tray and place the garlic slices on top. Sprinkle with the rosemary and drizzle with olive oil. Cover loosely with foil and roast for 25–30 minutes, turning halfway through.

Meanwhile, place the potatoes in a saucepan and cover with water. Bring to the boil and cook for 15 minutes or until the potatoes are soft. Drain, then add the milk and butter before mashing with a fork or potato masher.

Place the broccolini in a heatproof bowl and cover with boiling water. Leave for 3 minutes, then drain and refresh. Serve the lamb cutlets over mashed potato with the side of broccolini.

Serves 2

Chicken herb skewers with roast veggies

1 clove garlic, peeled
zest of ½ lemon
¼ cup basil leaves
2 teaspoons oregano leaves
¼ cup chopped flat-leaf parsley
200 g chicken breast, cut into 4 cm pieces
1 potato, cut into quarters
200 g pumpkin, cubed
1 onion, halved
1 carrot, cubed
olive oil, for drizzling
sea salt and black pepper

Crush the garlic, lemon zest, basil, oregano and parsley using a mortar and pestle. Transfer to a container with the chicken pieces and combine. Cover and place in the fridge for 30 minutes.

Preheat the oven to 220°C (200°C fan-forced).

Thread the chicken onto skewers and place on a baking tray. Lightly drizzle with oil and cover with foil. Roast for 20 minutes, then remove the foil and cook for another 10 minutes until the chicken is browned and cooked through.

Place the potato, pumpkin, onion and carrot in a roasting tin and lightly drizzle with oil. Season with salt and pepper and cover with foil. Roast for 20–30 minutes or until tender.

Serve the roast veg with the chicken skewers.

Serves 2

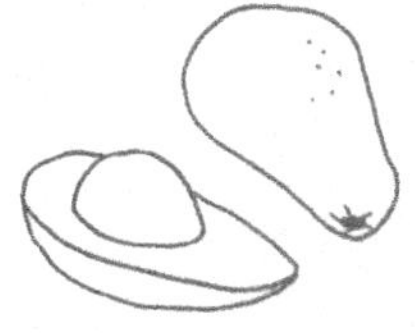

Tuna fishcakes

1 sweet potato, chopped
1 × 185 g can tuna, drained
1 free-range egg, whisked
½ cup quinoa flakes
¼ cup chopped spring onion
¼ cup chopped dill
zest and juice of ½ lemon
sea salt and black pepper
2 tablespoons olive oil
2 cups lettuce
1 cucumber, sliced
1 avocado, sliced

Preheat the oven to 200°C (180°C fan-forced) and line a baking tray with baking paper.

Place the sweet potato in a small saucepan and cover with water. Bring to the boil and cook for 10–15 minutes or until the sweet potato is tender. Drain, then mash with a fork.

Add the tuna, egg, quinoa flakes, spring onion, dill and lemon zest to the mashed sweet potato. Season with salt and pepper. Gently combine. Roll the mixture into small patties in the palm of your hand.

Place the fishcakes on the prepared tray and drizzle with 1 tablespoon of the olive oil. Bake for 10 minutes, then flip over and cook for another 10 minutes or until lightly browned on both sides.

Serve with a green salad of lettuce, cucumber and avocado, simply dressed with the remaining olive oil and the lemon juice.

Serves 2

Fettuccine bolognese

1 tablespoon olive oil
1 onion, diced
1 clove garlic, crushed
400 g lean mince
2 mushrooms, diced
1 carrot, diced
1 zucchini, diced
400 g can diced tomatoes
1 teaspoon pesto
175 g fettuccine
shaved parmesan, to serve

Heat the olive oil in a saucepan over medium heat and fry the onion and garlic for 1–2 minutes or until the onion is translucent. Add the mince and fry until browned. Add the mushroom, carrot, zucchini and tomatoes, then reduce the heat and cook, stirring, for 5 minutes. Stir through the pesto, then cover with a lid and simmer for 10–15 minutes.

Meanwhile, cook the fettuccine in boiling water according to the packet instructions.

Serve the pasta with the bolognese sauce and shaved parmesan.

Serves 2

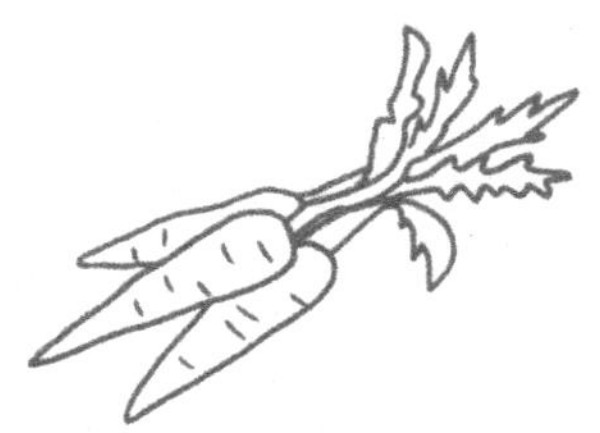

Stuffed baked potatoes

2 large brushed potatoes
100 g cottage cheese
1 small raw beetroot, cut into matchsticks
1 small carrot, cut into matchsticks
1 cup finely sliced red cabbage
1 avocado, sliced
1 apple, finely grated
1 tomato, diced

Preheat the oven to 200°C (180°C fan-forced).

Place the potatoes in a large saucepan and cover with water. Bring to the boil and cook for 10 minutes until par-boiled. Drain, then transfer to a baking tray and bake for 20 minutes, or until tender.

Make a lengthways cut in each baked potato. Fill with cottage cheese and finely sliced veg, then top with avocado, apple and tomato.

Serves 2

Romesco lamb chops & sweet potato

1 sweet potato, finely sliced
olive oil, for drizzling
2 lamb chops
10 green beans

Romesco sauce

185 g jar chargrilled capsicum, drained
¼ cup flaked almonds
1 clove garlic, peeled
1 tablespoon red wine vinegar
2 teaspoons smoked paprika
¼ cup chopped flat-leaf parsley

Preheat the oven to 200°C (180°C fan-forced).

To make the romesco sauce, place the ingredients in a food processor and blend until smooth.

Place the sweet potato on a baking tray and drizzle with oil. Cook for 15–20 minutes or until tender.

Meanwhile, place the lamb chops on a baking tray and bake for 5 minutes, then turn over and bake for another 5–10 minutes or until tender and well done.

Place the beans in a heatproof bowl and cover with boiling water. Leave for 3 minutes, then drain and refresh.

Serve the lamb and sweet potato with the romesco sauce and the green beans.

Serves 2

THANK YOU

Ruby

For the strongest woman I know: my nan, Pamela Gibb. The one who set the standard for all the women in my family, with her love, courage, commitment, sacrifice and her cheeky smile. To my mother and father, thank you for your support, love and kindness. My best friend and husband, Ben, thank you for your unwavering love and encouragement, always. My little guy Alby: I submitted my first draft the night before you were born – you are my little ray of sunshine. Quinn Minnie, you taught me to love unconditionally, to be patient and selfless. Thanks also to my pa, Doug; my brothers, Jack and Charlie; and my sister, Jane.

Thank you to David for bringing my baby into the world safely and coming on this journey with me.

Thank you to the incredibly talented team at Pan Macmillan. I will be forever grateful for your support and guidance, and for making this book a reality. Special mention to Ingrid Ohlsson, Ariane Durkin, Libby Turner, Kirby Armstrong, Charlotte Ree, Tracey Cheetham, Naomi van Groll, Megan Pigott and Miriam Cannell.

From the beginning, I had such an amazing community share their stories and answer my questions. Thank you Neil and Sue, Tai and Lynda, Monika, Erin K, Nadja, Hannah D, Olivia, Gill, Lauren, Kate M, Phoebe and Charlie C for your contributions and support.

David

To my wife, Cherie, who made our babies and contributed so much to this book. Thank you for being there for me, always, and helping me to understand the experience of pregnancy, labour and birth.

And my patients, past and present, who taught me all the rest and still find ways to surprise me.

RESOURCES

The Royal Women's Hospital
Informative fact sheets about pregnancy, labour and birth.
thewomens.org.au

Raising Children Network
Parenting website covering topics from pregnancy through to teens.
raisingchildren.net.au

COPE (Centre of Perinatal Excellence)
Information and advice on the emotional challenges of becoming and being a parent.
cope.org.au

The Gidget Foundation
Awareness programs and support services for perinatal anxiety and depression.
gidgetfoundation.org.au

Beyond Blue
Support for anxiety, depression and suicide prevention, with a helpline and online chat for new parents.
beyondblue.org.au

PANDA: Perinatal Anxiety and Depression Australia
Support, fact sheets and resources.
panda.org.au
National helpline: 1300 726 306

Australian Breastfeeding Association
Australia's leading authority on breastfeeding.
breastfeeding.asn.au
National helpline: 1800 686 268

EARLY PARENTING SERVICES:

NSW
tresillian.org.au
Baby advice and parenting tips.

karitane.com.au
Parenting services from birth to 5.

VIC
education.vic.gov.au
Practical information for Victorian parents and carers.

QLD
childrens.health.qld.gov.au
Fact sheets and support services.

ACT
Canberra Mothercraft Society
cmsinc.org.au
Support and health care for families of young children.

SA
Women's and Children's Health Network
cyh.com
Pregnancy, parenting and kids' health advice.

WA
ngala.com.au
Parenting, family, children and youth support.

TAS
dhhs.tas.gov.au
Child health and parenting services.

INDEX

First published 2019 in Macmillan
by Pan Macmillan Australia Pty Limited
1 Market Street, Sydney, New South Wales
Australia 2000

A CIP catalogue record for this book is available
from the National Library of Australia
http://catalogue.nla.gov.au

Text design by Kirby Armstrong
Typeset in 11pt Times New Roman by Midland Typesetters
Printed in Australia by IVE Group Australia Pty Ltd

The publishers and their respective employees or agents will not accept responsibility for injuries or damage occasioned to any person as a result of participation in the activities described in this book. It is recommended that individually tailored advice is sought from your healthcare professional.

We advise that the information contained in this book does not negate personal responsibility on the part of the reader for their own health and safety. It is recommended that individually tailored advice is sought from your healthcare or medical professional. The publishers and their respective employees, agents and authors are not liable for injuries or damage occasioned to any person as a result of reading or following the information contained in this book.

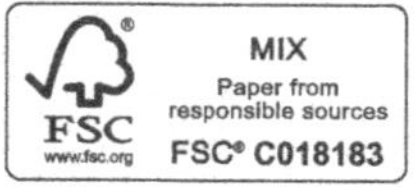

The paper in this book is FSC® certified.
FSC® promotes environmentally responsible, socially beneficial and economically viable management of the world's forests.